Lidija Cakarova

Alveolar Epithelial Repair in Gram Negative Bacterial Pneumonia

Lidija Cakarova

Alveolar Epithelial Repair in Gram Negative Bacterial Pneumonia

Macrophage-epithelial crosstalk during alveolar epithelial repair following pathogen-induced pulmonary inflammation

Südwestdeutscher Verlag für Hochschulschriften

Impressum / Imprint
Bibliografische Information der Deutschen Nationalbibliothek: Die Deutsche Nationalbibliothek verzeichnet diese Publikation in der Deutschen Nationalbibliografie; detaillierte bibliografische Daten sind im Internet über http://dnb.d-nb.de abrufbar.
Alle in diesem Buch genannten Marken und Produktnamen unterliegen warenzeichen-, marken- oder patentrechtlichem Schutz bzw. sind Warenzeichen oder eingetragene Warenzeichen der jeweiligen Inhaber. Die Wiedergabe von Marken, Produktnamen, Gebrauchsnamen, Handelsnamen, Warenbezeichnungen u.s.w. in diesem Werk berechtigt auch ohne besondere Kennzeichnung nicht zu der Annahme, dass solche Namen im Sinne der Warenzeichen- und Markenschutzgesetzgebung als frei zu betrachten wären und daher von jedermann benutzt werden dürften.

Bibliographic information published by the Deutsche Nationalbibliothek: The Deutsche Nationalbibliothek lists this publication in the Deutsche Nationalbibliografie; detailed bibliographic data are available in the Internet at http://dnb.d-nb.de.
Any brand names and product names mentioned in this book are subject to trademark, brand or patent protection and are trademarks or registered trademarks of their respective holders. The use of brand names, product names, common names, trade names, product descriptions etc. even without a particular marking in this work is in no way to be construed to mean that such names may be regarded as unrestricted in respect of trademark and brand protection legislation and could thus be used by anyone.

Verlag / Publisher:
Südwestdeutscher Verlag für Hochschulschriften
ist ein Imprint der / is a trademark of
OmniScriptum GmbH & Co. KG
Heinrich-Böcking-Str. 6-8, 66121 Saarbrücken, Deutschland / Germany
Email: info@svh-verlag.de

Herstellung: siehe letzte Seite /
Printed at: see last page
ISBN: 978-3-8381-1186-5

Zugl. / Approved by: Giessen, JLU, Diss., 2009

Copyright © 2009 OmniScriptum GmbH & Co. KG
Alle Rechte vorbehalten. / All rights reserved. Saarbrücken 2009

I. Table of Contents

I.	Table of Contents		1
II.	List of Figures		4
III.	Abbreviations		6
1.	Introduction		9
	1.1.	Pulmonary alveolus	9
	1.1.1.	Alveolar Epithelial Cells (AEC)	9
	1.1.2.	Resident alveolar macrophages (AMφ) – the sentinel phagocytic cell of the innate immune system of the lung	12
	1.2.	Pathogen-induced acute lung injury	12
	1.3.	Resolution of inflammation	14
	1.4.	Alveolar epithelial repair	15
	1.4.1.	Macrophage-epithelial crosstalk during alveolar epithelial repair	16
	1.4.2.	Granulocyte-macrophage colony-stimulating factor (GM-CSF)	18
	1.5.	*Klebsiella pneumoniae*	19
2.	Aims of the study		20
3.	Material and Methods		21
	3.1.	Animals	21
	3.2.	Isolation and culture of murine primary alveolar epithelial cells and preparation of lung homogenates	21
	3.3.	Isolation and culture of murine primary resident alveolar macrophages	22
	3.4.	AEC/AMφ *in vitro* co-culture	22
	3.5.	Gene expression analysis	23
	3.5.1.	Isolation of total RNA	23
	3.5.2.	cDNA synthesis	23
	3.5.3.	Real-time quantitative PCR (qPCR)	24
	3.6.	Protein expression analysis	25
	3.6.1.	Immunofluorescence	25
	3.6.2.	Flow cytometry	26
	3.6.3.	Western Blot	26
	3.6.4.	Cytokine quantification	28
	3.7.	*In vitro* proliferation assays	29
	3.7.1.	[^{3}H]-thymidine incorporation	29
	3.7.2.	Cell counting	29

3.8.	*In vivo* mouse treatment protocols	29
3.9.	Collection and analysis of blood samples and bronchoalveolar lavage fluid (BALF)	30
3.9.1.	Pappenheim-stained cytocentrifuge preparations	30
3.10.	*In vivo* lung permeability assay	31
3.11.	Measurement of *in vivo* proliferation of AEC II	31
3.11.1.	Total AEC numbers in lung homogenates	31
3.12.	Infection experiments with *K. pneumoniae*	32
4. Results		33
4.1.	LPS-stimulation of AMφ induces AEC growth factors in co-culture	33
4.2.	Epithelial GM-CSF expression is induced by alveolar macrophage TNF-α	35
4.3.	GM-CSF receptor expression is associated with the AEC II phenotype	38
4.4.	GM-CSF signalling in AEC	40
4.4.1.	GM-CSF stimulation is not associated with pro-inflammatory cytokine production in AEC	40
4.4.2.	AEC do not produce growth factors upon GM-CSF treatment	40
4.4.3.	GM-CSF induces proliferative signalling in AEC	41
4.5.	AEC proliferation is induced by macrophage TNF-α and mediated by GM-CSF	44
4.6.	TNF-α mediates AEC II proliferation following LPS-induced lung injury *in vivo*	45
4.7.	GM-CSF enhances AEC II proliferation and alveolar barrier renewal after LPS-induced acute lung injury	47
5. Discussion		54
5.1.	The contribution of pro-inflammatory resident alveolar macrophages to epithelial repair	55
5.2.	GM-CSF induced proliferative signalling in AEC	56
5.3.	The role of the TNF-α – GM-CSF axis in alveolar repair following acute lung injury	57
6. Summary		60
7. Zusammenfassung		62
8. References		64
9. Supplements		72
9.1.	Materials and source of supply	72

9.2.	Technical equipment and manufacturer	75
9.3.	List of primers for real-time RT-PCR	77
10.	Acknowledgements	78

II. List of Figures

Figure 1. The Normal Alveolus and the Injured Alveolus in the Acute Phase of Acute Lung Injury...............14
Figure 2. Epithelial cell repair following acute lung injury...............16
Figure 3. Regulation of macrophage activation by interaction with apoptotic cells...............17
Figure 4. A scheme of the *in vitro* co-culture model of primary murine AEC and AMϕ...............23
Figure 5. LPS-stimulated AMϕ enhance the expression of growth factors in co-cultured AEC...............34
Figure 6. GM-CSF secretion in the supernatants from AEC/AMϕ co-culture...............35
Figure 7. Quantification of TNF-α levels in AEC/AMϕ co-culture...............36
Figure 8. Expression of TNF-α receptors during AEC *in vitro* culture...............36
Figure 9. Alveolar macrophage TNF-α mediates epithelial GM-CSF production...............37
Figure 10. Recombinant TNF-α induces GM-CSF production in AEC *in vitro*...............37
Figure 11. Freshly isolated AEC express both GM-CSF receptor subunits...............38
Figure 12. Expression changes of the markers of type II and type I AEC phenotype during 5 days of culture of untreated or GM-CSF-treated AEC...............39
Figure 13. GM-CSF does not induce the release of pro-inflammatory chemokines in AEC...40
Figure 14. GM-CSF induces STAT5 phosphorylation in AEC...............41
Figure 15. Cyclin D1 mRNA expression is upregulated upon GM-CSF stimulation of AEC. 42
Figure 16. GM-CSF induces increased AEC proliferation...............42
Figure 17. Matrigel:collagen culture delays *in vitro* differentiation of murine AEC...............43
Figure 18. Matrigel:collagen cultured AEC express GM-CSF in co-culture with LPS stimulated AMϕ and proliferate upon GM-CSF stimulation...............44
Figure 19. GM-CSF mediates macrophage TNF-α induced AEC proliferation...............45
Figure 20. TNF-α mediates AEC II proliferation *in vivo*...............46
Figure 21. Neutralization of alveolar TNF-α reduces alveolar GM-CSF release after LPS challenge...............47
Figure 22. Quantification of total leukocyte numbers in BALF...............47
Figure 23. Quantification of BALF leukocyte subpopulations from Pappenheim-stained cytocentrifuged preparations...............48
Figure 24. TNF-α and GM-CSF levels in BAL fluid from LPS-treated mice...............49

Figure 25. GM-CSF-deficiency is associated with decreased AEC II proliferation after LPS-induced lung injury. 50

Figure 26. Reduction of total AEC numbers after LPS-induced lung injury is due to loss of AEC II but not of AEC I. 50

Figure 27. Alveolar leakage in wt (white bars), $GM^{-/-}$ (grey bars) and SPC-GM (black bars) at various time intervals post LPS administration. 51

Figure 28. Quantification of total BALF leukocytes and leukocyte-subpopulations after *K. pneumoniae* infection in wt mice. 52

Figure 29. TNF-α and GM-CSF levels in BALF from *K. pneumoniae* infected wt mice. 52

Figure 30. Alveolar repair after *K. pneumoniae* infection is associated with TNF-α-dependent AEC II proliferation. 53

Figure 31. Proposed model of AMϕ/AEC cross-talk in alveolar barrier repair. 54

III. Abbreviations

AEC	alveolar epithelial cells
ALI	acute lung injury
AMϕ	resident alveolar macrophages
APS	amonium persulfate
Aqp5	aquaporin 5
ARDS	acute respiratory distress syndrome
BAL(F)	bronchoalveolar lavage (fluid)
C/EBPα	CCAAT enhancer binding protein alpha
CCL2	CC chemokine ligand 2
CD	cluster of differentiation
CFU	colony forming units
DAPI	4', 6'- diamidino-2-phenylindole
DC	dendritic cells
dNTP	deoxynucleotide triphosphate
DTT	dithiothreitol
EGF	epidermal growth factor
ExMϕ	Exudate alveolar macrophages
FGF	fibroblast growth factor
GABRP	gamma amino-butyric acid pi-subunit
GM-CSF	granulocyte-macrophage colony stimulating factor
HGF	hepatocyte growth factor
HMBS	hydroxymethylbilane synthase
hpi	hours post infection

IGF 1/2	insulin-like growth factor 1/2
IL	interleukin
im	intramuscular
JAK-2	Janus kinase 2
KGF	keratinocyte growth factor
LPS	lypopolysaccharide
MAPK	mitogen-activated protein kinase
MIP-2	macrophage inflammatory protein 2
NF-κB	nuclear factor - κB
PAP	pulmonary alveolar proteinosis
PCR	polymerase chain reaction
PDGF	platelet derived growth factor
PGE2	prostaglandin E2
rpm	rounds per minute
RT	room temperature
SD	standard deviation
SDS	sodium dodecyl-sulphate
SP	surfactant proteins
STAT	signal transducer and activator of transcription
TGF α/β	transforming growth factor alpha/beta
TLR-4	Toll-like receptor-4
TNF-α	tumour necrosis factor - alpha
VEGF	vascular endothelial growth factor
WSCK	Wide spread cytokeratin
wt	wild type

1. Introduction

1.1. Pulmonary alveolus

The lung is a specialized organ for gas exchange and represents the largest epithelial surface of the body in contact with the external environment. It is consisted of the two functionally and structurally distinct regions known as upper (or proximal, conducting) and lower (or distal) respiratory tracts. The upper respiratory tract (nose, pharynx) serves to filter, warm and humidify inhaled air, thus protecting the respiratory membranes of the lower tract from damage. The trachea connects the upper to the lower respiratory tract which further divides into left and right main bronchi. The main bronchi are often considered as the start of the lower respiratory tract, functioning in the conduction of inspired air through to the gas exchange region of the alveoli. Further bifurcations of the bronchi lead to formation of small bronchi, bronchioles and terminal bronchioles. The far distal respiratory zone ultimately comprises the respiratory bronchioles, alveolar ducts, and the alveoli themselves (1).

The alveoli, or air sacs, are organized as clusters continuous with the alveolar ducts. Each pulmonary alveolus is surrounded by many blood capillaries constituting an extensive air–blood interface, comprised mainly of alveolar epithelium and pulmonary capillary endothelium, which allows an optimal gas-diffusion across the respiratory membrane. The alveolar epithelial surface is covered with a film of surfactant that lowers the surface tension in the lungs and is essential when the alveolar sacs are to expand during inspiration (1, 2).

The interstitium lying between the alveolar epithelium and pulmonary capillary endothelium is made up of several different cell types (fibroblasts, mast cells, myofibroblasts and dendritic cells) and basement membrane components (1, 3). The alveolar wall itself is consisted of two main cell types: alveolar epithelial cells and resident alveolar macrophages (Fig. 1).

1.1.1. Alveolar Epithelial Cells (AEC)

Alveolar epithelium is comprised of two morphologically and functionally distinct cell types, alveolar epithelial cells type I (AEC I) and type II (AEC II) (Fig. 1). Highly flattened AEC I cover 95% of the internal alveolar surface area, whereas cuboidal AEC II cover the remaining 5%.

A major function of AEC II is the synthesis of surfactant (surface active agent) and its subsequent release from the intracellular storage granules (lamellar bodies) by exocytosis upon different stimuli (4). Its primary role is to provide efficient ventilation by regulating

Introduction

surface tension according to the alveolar size. Surfactant is composed of 90% phospholipids and 10% proteins (surfactant proteins (SP) -A, B, C and D). Although a few other lung cells may produce SP-A, SP-B and SP-D, AEC II are the only pulmonary cells known to produce all surfactant components. SP-C is known to be produced only by AEC II (5-7).

Studies investigating the mechanisms of pulmonary oedema clearance revealed that the alveolar barrier is not just a tight epithelium but it also participates in the active ion and solute transport across the epithelial-endothelial barrier (8). Hence, AEC II are known to possess membrane bound water channels and ion pumps, enabling them to form a very thin aqueous film (hypophase), which serves as an environment for extracellular biochemical reactions as well as a "medium" for intra-alveolar cells such as resident alveolar macrophages and enables paracrine cellular crosstalk via soluble mediators (6, 9, 10).

AEC II have been shown to have unlimited potential for proliferation and self-renewal, and are therefore described as the stem cell of the alveolar epithelium (6, 11-14). Hence, the following concept for AEC II as the alveolar stem cell, as well as the process of transition of AEC II into AEC I following injury, was postulated (15): upon lung injury the nearest AEC II proliferate and, if necessary, differentiate into squamous AEC I, which are terminally differentiated and thus incapable of division. However, only a fraction of the daughter cells differentiate; the remaining part is believed to retain type II phenotype thereby replenishing the original stem cell population. Transition into AEC I may be preceded by division of AEC II (differentiation) or may occur without any mitotic events (trans-differentiation). The *in vivo* evidence for the process of differentiation/trans-differentiation are obscure; however numerous *in vitro* studies supported this concept, as described in details in the next section (*1.1.1.1 AEC in vitro culture*). Of note, emerging evidence suggests the possibility that not all AEC II in the lung, but a certain subpopulation has the capacity to repopulate the injured epithelium (15-17).

AEC I compose the largest part of the peripheral lung and due to their morphology are highly specialized cells for gas exchange. In contrast to AEC II, the biology of AEC I has been largely unexplored, because until recently it has been impossible to isolate these fragile cells from the lungs and to culture them *in vitro*. AEC I have numerous cellular extensions which occasionally may form the epithelium of more than one alveolus, thereby building a complex architecture which partially explains their greater susceptibility to injury (14, 18, 19).

Another difficulty accompanying the AEC I research is the deficiency of specific cellular markers for these cells. T1-α (podoplanin, gp 38, RTI 40) has been described as the first and most reliable marker for AEC I and its expression in the adult lung has been restricted to type I cells (14, 18, 20).

AEC I expression of aquaporin 5 (Aqp-5) (14, 21), a member of the water channels family, and the phenotype of Aqp-5 knock-out mice indicated that AEC I are competent cells for ion and water transport. A recent study (22) clearly evidenced that rat AEC I express Na^+, K^+ channels and cystic fibrosis trans-membrane regulator (CFTR), thereby supporting this hypothesis.

1.1.1.1. AEC *in vitro* culture

Primary culture of alveolar epithelial cells, particularly AEC II, is a widely accepted model for studying their biology. According to the common paradigm, AEC II over several days of *in vitro* culture differentiate/ trans-differentiate into AEC I-like cells, a process which resembles the AEC II *in vivo* differentiation. This concept was postulated in 1992 in the study from Shannon *et al.* (23) showing that rat AEC II cultured on fibroblast feeder layers lose their lamellar bodies and acquire specific AEC I morphology. Similarly, Danto *et al.* provided evidence that differentiated AEC II grown on collagen gels acquire additional AEC I specific antigens.

Over the next 15 years numerous studies further developed these *in vitro* concepts; the majority of them emphasizing the influence of the culture conditions on AEC differentiation. Hence, keratinocyte growth factor (KGF) prevents increase of T1-α expression in rat AEC II cultures (24), thereby promoting *in vitro* maintenance of the type II phenotype. Likewise, the matrigel:collagen culture substrate enables phenotype preservation of murine and human alveolar epithelial type II cells (25, 26).

Despite the numerous evidence supporting the concept of AEC II to I differentiation, the molecular signals underlying these phenotype changes (*in vivo* and *in vitro*) remain largely unknown. Transforming growth factor-ß1 (TGF-ß1) is the only molecule shown to be involved in AEC II to AEC I *in vitro* differentiation (27), whereas c-Jun N-terminal kinase (JNK) has been shown to mediate KGF-induced preservation of AEC II phenotype (28).

However, given that the isolation of AEC I has been recently established only in rats, and is associated with low yields (29), AEC I-like cells differentiated over 5-7 days from AEC II remain to be a reliable model of lung alveolar type I epithelial cells.

Introduction

1.1.2. Resident alveolar macrophages (AMφ) – the sentinel phagocytic cell of the innate immune system of the lung

A large array of microbial products and particles enter the lungs on a daily basis. Contaminants larger in size either deposit in the upper respiratory tract or sediment on its mucociliary surface, thereby being prevented from further spread into the alveolar space. Contaminants smaller then 1 μm, such as bacteria and viral particles, are carried to the alveolar surface where they interact with local innate immune system components - alveolar fluids (e.g. IgA, complement, surfactants) and resident leukocytes. Normally, resident alveolar macrophages (AMφ) account for ~ 95% of airspace leukocytes, with 1 to 4% lymphocytes and only about 1% neutrophils, thereby representing the major sentinel phagocytic cell of the innate immune system of the lungs (30). Resident alveolar macrophages are known to form the first line of defence against bacteria invading the alveolar air space. They are distributed at the air-tissue interface of the alveolar space and closely adhere to alveolar epithelial cells.

Though AMφ are avidly phagocytic and ingest large numbers of particles, they are relatively inert in terms of triggering inflammatory responses because their primary role is to keep airspaces quiescent. However, when the microbial challenge is too numerous or too virulent to be contained by macrophages alone, AMφ mount an innate immune response and local inflammation (30, 31).

1.2. Pathogen-induced acute lung injury

Acute lung injury (ALI) and its severest form acute respiratory distress syndrome (ARDS) are definitions of acute respiratory failure, caused by diffuse damage to the pulmonary parenchyma within hours to days by a variety of local or systemic insults (32). Increased alveolar-capillary membrane permeability due to endothelial and epithelial disruption and/or diffuse inflammatory reaction in the pulmonary parenchyma, was recognized as the common end of organ injury and a central feature in all forms of ALI/ARDS (33). Due to the increased permeability of the alveolar–capillary barrier, an extensive extravasation of protein-rich fluid into the air spaces takes place, which consequently leads to a formation of pulmonary oedema. Alveolar epithelial damage in ALI is associated with impaired lung ion/water transport and subsequent clearance of the edema fluid, as well as surfactant abnormalities. Moreover, disrupted epithelium may result in a septic shock in patients with pneumonia due to translocation of pathogens into the blood stream, and finally persistent severe injury without organized and sufficient epithelial repair may lead to lung fibrosis (34).

Introduction

Alveolar microbial challenge leads to activation of AMφ and subsequent release of pro-inflammatory cytokines that are under the control of the transcription factors of the nuclear factor-κB family (NF-κB). These cytokines are interleukin (IL)-1β, tumour necrosis factor (TNF)-α, IL-6, IL-12, macrophage inhibitory protein (MIP) – 1α. TNF-α and IL-1ß are designated as early response cytokines (35) and stimulate production of chemo-attractants from epithelial cells, such as macrophage inflammatory protein (MIP)-2 (the most potent neutrophil attractant) and CCL2 (monocyte attractant) in mice (31, 36, 37). Furthermore TNF-α induces up-regulation of adhesion molecules, thereby enhancing neutrophil influx from the surrounding blood capillary in the alveolar space. Apart from the production of pro-inflammatory cytokines, AMφ directly ingest pathogens, and both AMφ and recruited neutrophils have receptors for antibodies and complement, so that the coating of microorganisms with antibodies, complement, or both, enhances phagocytosis. The engulfed microorganisms are subjected to a wide range of toxic intracellular molecules, including superoxide anion, hydroxyl radicals, hypochlorous acid, nitric oxide, antimicrobial cationic proteins and peptides, and lysozyme. Phagocytes also remove the body's own dead or dying cells, thereby preventing further development of the inflammatory reactions at the site of injury (38).

During the later course of inflammation the destroyed AMφ pool in the alveolar space is replaced by lung-differentiation of peripheral blood monocytes ("exudate macrophages", ExMφ). ARDS has been associated with high levels of the chemokine CCL2, the major monocyte chemoattractant (39).

AEC are active participants in the inflammatory reaction and respond to the presence of microbes by induction of two complementary parts of an innate immune response: 1) increased production of antimicrobial agents and 2) induction of a signal network to recruit leukocytes (40). Hence SP-A and SP-D act as collectins, opsonize the pathogen and allow phagocytosis by AMφ. Furthermore, AEC express a variety of toll-like receptors for pathogen recognition and in response to LPS have been shown to produce chemokines and the potent antimicrobial peptide human ß-defensin-2 (HBD2) and LPS-neutralizing peptide LL-37 (cathelicidin) (41, 42). During Influenza virus infection CCL2 is strongly released from murine AEC, thereby stimulating remarkable monocyte transmigration across the epithelium. (43).

Pathogen-induced tissue damage, massive inflammatory responses and dying alveolar cells lead to acute lung injury and require ultimate resolution of inflammation to restore normal lung function.

Introduction

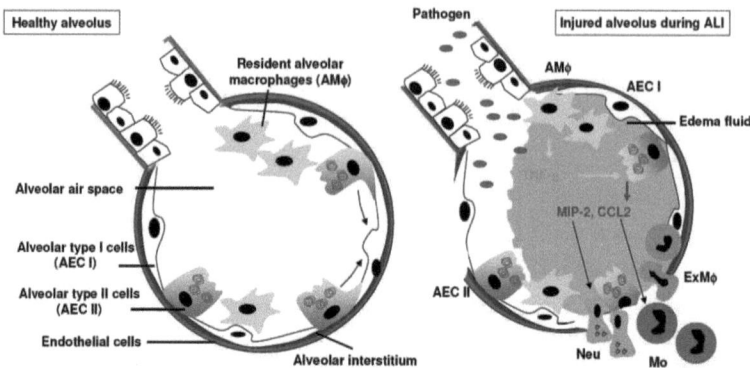

Figure 1. The Normal Alveolus and the Injured Alveolus in the Acute Phase of Acute Lung Injury. *Left panel:* Healthy alveolus in steady state represents a quiescent environment, composed of the following structures: the alveolar wall structured by alveolar epithelial cells (AEC II and AEC I), resident alveolar macrophages (AMϕ), the alveolar endothelium and the alveolar interstitium. *Right panel:* Following pathogen invasion AMϕ are the first cells to respond and secrete TNF-α, which acts locally to stimulate production of pro-inflammatory cytokines by AEC such as MIP-2 and CCL2, thereby stimulating rapid neutrophil (Neu) influx into the alveolar space, followed by monocyte (Mo) recruitment from the surrounding capillaries. Once they reach the alveolar space Mo differentiate into macrophages (exudate macrophages, ExMϕ). Consequently, the pathogen itself and the massive inflammation cause a severe damage to the sensitive endo-epithelial alveolar barrier, which finally leads to oedema formation and alveolar flooding. Neu, neutrophils: Mo, monocytes; ExMϕ, exudate macrophages.

1.3. Resolution of inflammation

Reestablishment of the tissue homeostasis (resolution) is a complex and actively regulated process that involves all resident alveolar cells (44).

Neutrophils recruited in the alveolar space after microbial invasion neutralise and eliminate the injurious stimuli. This step, though obvious, is perhaps the critical one for acute inflammation to resolve. Hence, phagocyte removal of the pathogens, accompanied with release of factors that prevent ongoing neutrophil trafficking and oedema formation represent the first step in resolution of acute inflammation (45). The second and most important step in resolution is disposal of the neutrophils from the site of injury in a controlled and effective manner, to protect the alveolus from further harm. Pro-inflammatory arachidonic acid products prostaglandin E2 and D2, released from neutrophils upon pathogen phagocytosis, stimulate the switch of arachidonic-acid-metabolism into production of the pro-resolution lipid mediators lipoxins, resolvins and protectins (44). Recent results indicate that, as inflammation proceeds, neutrophils in exudates stop producing chemoattractants and within hours begin to convert arachidonic acid into protective lipoxins (46, 47). Murine macrophages generate lipoxins upon engulfment of apoptotic leukocytes (48). Specific lipoxins, resolvins and protectins provide potent signals that selectively stop neutrophil infiltration, stimulate recruitment of monocytes (without elaborating pro-inflammatory mediators); activate macrophage phagocytosis of microorganisms and apoptotic cells; increase the exit of phagocytes from the inflamed site through the lymphatics, and stimulate the expression of molecules involved in antimicrobial defence (49, 50). The last, but equally important aspect of inflammation resolution is that parenchymal cells, which hosted the inflammatory event are reverted into a non-inflammatory phenotype and destroyed parenchymal cells are replaced (51).

1.4. Alveolar epithelial repair

The diffuse alveolar damage accompanying the acute phase of lung injury is ultimately followed by effective endo-epithelial barrier renewal to restore normal lung function. The most damaged structure is the alveolar type I cell, which appears to be more sensitive to injury then alveolar type II cells (11). Of note, endothelial cell damage is subtle and seems to be of minor importance in maintenance of alveolar barrier integrity. The key features of successful alveolar repair after ALI are oedema fluid clearance and reconstitution of a normal alveolar structure. Epithelial repair consists of proliferation and differentiation, adhesion, spreading and migration of alveolar epithelial cells. As described in *Section 1.1.1*. AEC II are a source of distal airway epithelial recovery. The daily turnover rate of AEC II is remarkably low at 4% but rapidly increases after injury (11). However, epithelial cell proliferation needs several hours to take place and 1-2 days to become significant (Fig. 2) (8).

Adhesion to the extracellular matrix, spreading and migration have been suggested to precede the epithelial proliferative phase. Hence, AEC II have been shown to migrate *in vitro* in response to different growth factors and cytokines, such as epidermal growth factor (EGF), transforming growth factor-alpha (TGF-α), laminin, fibronectin, and IL-1ß and TNF-α to a lesser extent. Interestingly AEC II do not need to be in a proliferative phase to exhibit increased motility (52). However, the *in vivo* contribution of AEC spreading and migration in epithelial repair has been poorly investigated due to the lack of sensitive tools to study these processes *in vivo*. Of note, while migration can take up to a few minutes for neutrophils, it needs several hours to be initiated in AEC (52).

Introduction

Both migration and proliferation of AEC require modulators. Heparin sulphate-binding cytokines – such as epidermal growth factor (EGF), hepatocyte growth factor (HGF), transforming growth factor alpha (TGF-α), keratinocyte growth factor (KGF), and fibroblast growth factor (FGF) were identified as promoters of epithelial cell migration and proliferation after lung injury (53-55).

Transforming growth factor beta (TGF-β) participates in alveolar repair by attenuating the inflammatory cytokine production from AMφ (56), enhancing production of matrix protein components (57) and regulating integrin expression on epithelial cells (58). Similarly, platelet derived growth factor (PDGF) is mitogenic for fetal alveolar epithelial cells (59), and it has been demonstrated to enhance DNA synthesis in adult rat alveolar epithelial cells (60).

Besides the soluble modulators, alveolar epithelial repair is tightly regulated by the cells neighbouring AEC in the alveolus, particularly resident alveolar macrophages. However, the molecular mechanisms underlying the crosstalk between AEC and the other resident alveolar cells during alveolar repair remain largely elusive.

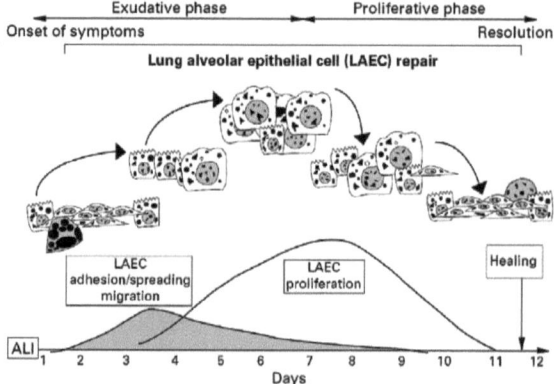

Figure 2. Epithelial cell repair following acute lung injury. The different stages involved in the process are illustrated. ALI = acute lung injury; LAEC = lung alveolar epithelial cell. Adapted from Berthiaume *et al.* 1999 (8).

1.4.1. Macrophage-epithelial crosstalk during alveolar epithelial repair

Resident alveolar macrophages are suggested to play a dual role in ALI. During the acute inflammatory phase AMφ acquire a pro-inflammatory phenotype engaged to dispose of the pathogens from the alveolar space, followed by the switch into an anti-inflammatory phenotype which initiates the resolution phase, as described in *Section 1.3*. The later AMφ phenotype has been associated with the release of epithelial growth factors and anti-inflammatory cytokines, and hence with the potential to enhance alveolar repair.

In this respect Morimoto *et al.* showed that AMφ ingesting apoptotic neutrophils *in vitro* produce significant amounts of the potent epithelial mitogen HGF (61). Similarly, Fadok *et al.* provided evidence that upon phagocytosis of apoptotic cells AMφ produce TGF-ß, PGE2 and platelet- activating factor (PAF) – anti-inflammatory cytokines which consequently dampen LPS-induced production of pro-inflammatory cytokines by AMφ (56, 62). These studies emphasize the potential of AMφ to acquire an anti-inflammatory, reparative phenotype during later stages of inflammation, i.e. upon contact with apoptotic neutrophils or host cells (Fig. 3).

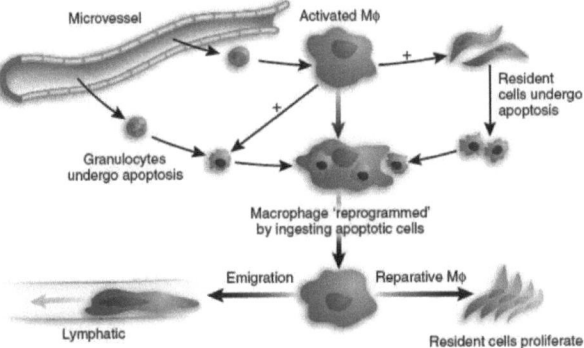

Figure 3. Regulation of macrophage activation by interaction with apoptotic cells. Activated macrophages (Mφ) can accelerate leukocyte apoptosis and trigger resident cell apoptosis. Subsequent phagocytosis of the apoptotic progeny deactivates or 'reprograms' the macrophage, which then receives signals to promote repair and/or emigrate. Adapted from Serhan 2005, (63).

Interestingly, several reports evidenced that AMφ may promote epithelial repair irrespectively of the contact with apoptotic cells. In this line, supernatants from silica-exposed AMφ increased DNA synthesis in AEC II *in vitro* via macrophage soluble mediators such as PDGF-like and IGF-like molecules (60). Furthermore, the macrophage pro-inflammatory cytokine IL-1ß enhanced *in vitro* epithelial repair by stimulating AEC spreading and migration via induction of TGF-α and EGF production in epithelial cells (64). TNF-α on the other hand stimulated *in vitro* proliferation of gastric epithelial cells by inducing arachidonic acid/prostaglandin pathway (65), whereas *in vivo* it has been demonstrated to enhance fluid clearance following bacterial pneumonia (66). Hence, the latter studies brought forward the notion that not only anti-inflammatory, but also the "early" pro-inflammatory AMɸ may contribute to epithelial repair; however the mechanisms need to be further investigated.

1.4.2. Granulocyte-macrophage colony-stimulating factor (GM-CSF)

Granulocyte macrophage colony-stimulating factor (GM-CSF) is produced by lung cells predominantly by alveolar macrophages and AEC II (67). It has been mainly recognized as a growth factor for the cells of the phagocytic lineage but also stimulates differentiation of eosinophils, erythrocytes, megakaryocytes and dendritic cells (68). Separately from its role in progenitor cell proliferation and differentiation, GM-CSF stimulates a number of functions of AMɸ, such as cytokine expression, killing of pathogens, surface receptor-antigen expression, adherence and oxidative metabolism (67).

The effects of GM-CSF are mediated through heteromeric cell-surface receptors. The GM-CSF receptor (GM-CSF R) is composed of low-affinity α (GM-CSF Rα) and high-affinity ß (GM-CSF Rß) chains (69, 70). Neither GM-CSF Rα nor GM-CSF Rß contains a tyrosine kinase catalytic domain but the ß chain constitutively associates with Janus kinase-2 (JAK-2), which is a tyrosine kinase (71). GM-CSF binds with the α-subunit, which then associates with the ß subunit and initiates JAK-2 phosphorylation and downstream signalling, such as activation of STAT or MAPK pathways (72).

Surprisingly, mice genetically deficient of GM-CSF ($GM^{-/-}$ mice) revealed a specific lung phenotype resembling to the human disease pulmonary alveolar proteinosis (PAP), which was found to be associated with AMɸ metabolic dysfunction. Therefore, GM-CSF has been assigned a crucial role in the surfactant homeostasis in healthy lungs (73, 74).

Furthermore, studies in transgenic mice created in the $GM^{-/-}$ background specifically overexpressing GM-CSF in AEC II (SPC-GM), revealed prominent hyperplasia and proliferation of AEC II (75), indicating these cells to be a GM-CSF target. Similarly, Joshi *et al.* demonstrated the expression of GM-CSF receptors on AEC II (76). Furthermore, GM-CSF exhibited epithelial protective effects after hyperoxic lung injury alone or associated with *Pneumocystis murina* pneumonia, such as preservation of the epithelial barrier, due to reduced alveolar wall cell apoptosis (77, 78). The aforementioned studies strengthened the notion that GM-CSF additionally targets other cells than phagocytes, such as AEC II, and hence may be involved in alveolar epithelial repair following ALI.

1.5. *Klebsiella pneumoniae*

Klebsiella pneumoniae is a gram-negative, encapsulated, facultative anaerobic bacterium; clinically the most important member of the *Klebsiella* genus of Enterobacteriaceae. It is ubiquitous and hence naturally occurs in the soil, and in the normal flora of the mouth, skin, and intestines in humans (79). *K. pneumoniae* causes severe pneumonia and frequently affects immunocompromized patients and alcoholics. *Klebsiellae* are also important in nosocomial infections among adult and paediatric populations, and account for approximately 8% of all hospital-acquired infections. In this line, outbreaks of *Klebsiellae* infections in neonatal units have been widely reported and are frequently associated with systemic infections, and death (80). This becomes increasingly important since an increasing number of nosocomial *K. pneumoniae* isolates are resistant to multiple antibiotics treatment. The infection is characterised by destructive changes, necrosis, inflammation, and haemorrhage within the lung tissue (81).

2. Aims of the study

In the presented thesis the following questions have been addressed:

1) Can early activated, pro-inflammatory resident alveolar macrophages initiate alveolar epithelial repair processes following lung inflammation?

2) What are the underlying molecular signals mediating macrophage-epithelial crosstalk during these processes, *in vitro* and *in vivo*?

To answer these questions an *in vitro* model of crosstalk between murine alveolar epithelial cells and lipopolysaccharide (LPS)–stimulated resident alveolar macrophages was established. Furthermore, LPS and *K. pneumoniae*-induced acute lung injury models were used to evaluate *in vivo* macrophage-epithelial crosstalk mechanisms involved in alveolar epithelial repair.

3. Material and Methods

3.1. Animals

Wild-type C57BL/6 mice (weight 18-21g) were purchased from Charles River (Sulzfeld, Germany). GM-CSF-deficient mice ($GM^{-/-}$) were produced by gene-targeting on a C57BL/6 background, as previously described (74). Transgenic mice overexpressing GM-CSF in AEC II were generated in $GM^{-/-}$ mice by expression of a chimeric gene containing GM-CSF under control of the human SP-C promoter, i.e. in AEC II (SPC-GM) (82). Both $GM^{-/-}$ and SPC-GM mice were a kind gift from Dr. Jeffrey Whitsett (University of Cincinnati, Ohio). Animals were kept under special pathogen-free conditions and used at 8-11 weeks of age. All animal experiments were approved by the local government committee of Giessen.

3.2. Isolation and culture of murine primary alveolar epithelial cells and preparation of lung homogenates

Type II AEC were isolated by the method developed by Corti *et al.* (83), with some modifications (43, 84). Briefly, lavaged and perfused lungs were filled with 1.5 ml sterile Dispase and 0.5 ml low-melting-point agarose (1%), removed and placed in Dispase for 40 min at room temperature. The lung parenchyma was subsequently teased from the airways and minced in DMEM/2.5% HEPES with 0.01% DNase, and successively passed through 100, 40, and 20 µm nylon filters. At this stage the lung homogenates were obtained in a form of single-cell suspension. The cell suspension was collected by centrifugation and incubated with biotinylated CD45, CD16/32 and CD31 to deplete leukocytes and endothelial cells, for 30 min. After washing, the contaminating cells were removed by incubation with streptavidin-linked magnetic particles, and subsequent magnetic separation. The supernatant was recovered and the purity of the AEC preparation was routinely assessed by flow cytometry. Final cell suspension always consisted of > 95% of AEC, i.e. pro-SP-C^+ cells. Viability was always >95%, as assessed by trypan blue dye exclusion. AECs stained positive for wide-spread cytokeratin (WSCK) throughout day 5 of culture as analysed by flow cytometry. For real-time PCR, Western Blot analysis, cytokine quantification and cell-counting the AEC were seeded in a 24-well cell-culture plate at a density of 2.5-5.0 x10^5 /well and cultured for up to 5 days. For [^{3}H]-thymidine-incorporation experiments 1.2 x10^5 AEC were seeded in a 48-well plate. For flow cytometry analysis AEC were grown on the lower side of the transwell filter inserts (6.4 mm diameter, 8 µm pore size) at a density of 3×10^5 and grown for up to 5 days.

For matrigel:collagen experiments freshly isolated AEC were seeded in a 24-well plate previously coated for 30 min with a 1:1 mixture of matrigel:collagen at a density of 4×10^5 cells/well. For mono-culture experiments AEC were left to attach for 5 h in medium containing 10% FCS, subsequently starved in medium with 0.1% FCS and cultured for up to 3 days. For proliferation analysis, after the initial 5 h attachment, AEC were stimulated with GM-CSF as indicated. The cells were removed from the matrigel:collagen matrix by 30 min incubation with 0.1% Collagenase A in Dispase solution at 37°C, and used for further applications.

AEC medium was composed of Dulbecco's MEM containing 4.5 g/l glucose, 12.5 mM HEPES, 2mM L-glutamine and penicillin/streptomycin.

Epithelial cells were kept in medium supplemented with 10% FCS for the first 16 to 24 h, and thereafter cultured in medium with 0.1% FCS (starving medium).

3.3. Isolation and culture of murine primary resident alveolar macrophages

Murine resident alveolar macrophages were isolated by bronchoalveolar lavage (BAL) from mouse lungs with sterile, ice-cold 2 mM PBS/EDTA. After centrifugation (1400 rpm, 10min), AMϕ were recovered in RPMI 1640 containing 10% FCS, 2mM L-glutamine and antibiotics. Before AEC/AMϕ co-culture experiments AMϕ seeded at a density of 2-2.5×10^5/well in a 24 well plate or on transwells were left to adhere for 1-2 h.

3.4. AEC/AMϕ *in vitro* co-culture

For AEC/AMϕ co-culture experiments, AEC were seeded on the lower side of transwells at a density of 3.0–5.0×10^5/well. For real-time PCR analysis and cytokine quantification AEC were grown on transwells for 60 h (70% confluence) in medium containing 10% FCS and then placed above the AMϕ grown in a 24 well plate (Fig. 4). Co-culture was maintained for the next 48 h, in 500 µl of AEC medium supplemented with 0.1% FCS. For [^{3}H]-thymidine-incorporation AEC were grown on transwells for 16 h in 10% FCS medium, starved for 10 h in 0.1% FCS medium and co-culture started immediately thereafter for 48 h. For matrigel:collagen co-culture experiments freshly isolated AEC were left to attach for 5 h in

Materials and Methods

medium containing 10% FCS, washed and immediately thereafter the co-culture with AMφ (grown on transwells) was started and maintained in starving medium (0.1% FCS) for 48-72 h.

In selected experiments, neutralizing anti-TNF-α or appropriate isotype IgG antibodies (1 µg/ml) were added to the medium of each AEC/AMφ co-culture-well at 0, 6, 12 and 20 h after LPS stimulation.

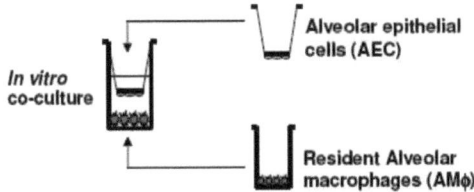

Figure 4. A scheme of the *in vitro* co-culture model of primary murine AEC and AMφ. AEC were grown on the lower side of the transwells and then co-cultured with primary AMφ for 48 h, with or without LPS.

3.5. Gene expression analysis

3.5.1. Isolation of total RNA

AEC and AMφ were lysed with TRK buffer and total cellular RNA was isolated with spin columns using PeqGold Total RNA kit. Subsequently, RNA was quantified by a spectrophotometer (Nanodrop ND-100). Total RNA from transwell co-cultured AEC was obtained by pooling the quantity from 3-5 transwells.

3.5.2. cDNA synthesis

After isolation mRNA was transcribed into cDNA by reverse transcriptase (RT) -reaction. To perform cDNA synthesis 50-500 ng of total RNA was mixed with water, heated for 5 min at 70° C, immediately thereafter transferred on ice and RT mix was added.

The total reaction volume was 25 µl. The mixture was then incubated for 1 h on 37° C, heated on 94° C for 7 min to inactivate the enzyme. The obtained cDNA was either used for real-time PCR or stored in -20° C until further use.

RT mix	Stock solution	Quantities per reaction
5x First strand buffer	250 mM Tris-HCl (pH 8.3), 375 mM KCl, 15 mM MgCl$_2$	5 µl
Random hexamers	100 ng/µl	150 ng
dNTPs	10 mM each	2.5 nmol each
DTT	100 mM	250 nmol
Ribonuclease inhibitor	40 U/µl	20 U
MMLV	200 U/µl	150 U

3.5.3. Real-time quantitative PCR (qPCR)

Quantitative gene expression analysis was performed by real-time PCR, using Platinum SYBR®Green qPCR SuperMix-UDG. DNA was detected and quantified with the fluorescent dye SYBR Green I which offers a linear dose response over a wide range of target concentrations, and binds directly to double-stranded (ds) DNA. As dsDNA accumulates the dye generates a signal that is proportional to the DNA concentration. ROX reference dye was used to normalize the fluorescent signal between reactions. PCR reactions were performed in 25 µl volume by using the qPCR mix.

qPCR mix	Stock solution	Quantities per reaction
SYBR®Green mix	2x (Taq DNA Polymerase, SYBR Green dye I, Tris-HCl, KCl, 6 mM MgCl2, 400 µM dGTP, dATP, dCTP, 800 µM dUTP, uracil DNA glycosylase, stabilizers)	13 µl
MgCl$_2$	50 mM	50 nmol
Forward primer	10 pmol/µl	5 pmol
Reverse primer	10 pmol/µl	5 pmol
H$_2$O	Molecular biology grade	5 µl
cDNA	2,5 ng/µl	12,5 ng

Cycling conditions were as follows: 95° C for 5 min, 45 cycles of 95° C for 10 s, 60° C for 30 s and 72° C for 10 s. Formation of a single specific PCR product was confirmed by melting curve analysis and agarose gel electrophoresis. Mouse hydroxymethylbilane synthase

(HMBS) served as a reference gene for all real-time PCR reactions. Relative changes in gene expression were determined with the ΔCt method using the following formula: $\Delta Ct = Ct_{reference} - Ct_{target}$. The oligonucleotide primer pairs used in qPCR were designed by Primer Express 2.0 and GenScript (https://www.genscript.com/ssl-bin/app/primer) programs. All primer sequences are listed in Supplement 9.3.

3.6. Protein expression analysis

3.6.1. Immunofluorescence

3.6.1.1. Immunofluorescence staining of cultured AEC

For immunofluorescence staining, AEC were either cultured on chamber-slides or on transwells. Prior to staining AEC were permeabilized and fixed in an ice-cold (-20°C) mixture of acetone and methanol (1:1) for 5 min, washed in 0.1% BSA/PBS and blocked with 3% BSA/PBS solution to prevent unspecific binding, until further antibody-staining. For primary antibody staining AEC were incubated overnight (anti-pro-SP-C and anti-T1-α antibodies, diluted 1:400 and 1:250, respectively) at 4°C, subsequently washed three times in 0.1% BSA/PBS (5 min each wash), and immediately thereafter incubated with Alexa 555-labelled anti rabbit IgG and Alexa 488-labelled anti hamster IgG secondary antibodies, (diluted in 0.1% BSA/PBS, 1:1000), for 1 h at RT. Secondary antibody excess was removed by three subsequent washes (in 0.1 % BSA/PBS, 5 min each). The slides were then mounted with Vectashield® mounting medium (containing DAPI for nuclear staining). Cells were imaged with conventional fluorescence microscopy using a Leica DM 2000 fluorescence microscope at the indicated magnification and Leica digital imaging software.

3.6.1.2. Immunofluorescence staining of lung tissue slices

Mouse lungs were perfused and lavaged with 500 µl 2mM EDTA/PBS aliquots to remove alveolar leukocytes, subsequently inflated with 1.5 ml of 1:1 mixture of TissueTek (Sakura) and PBS, removed en bloc and snap-frozen in liquid nitrogen. Lung tissue cryosections (7µm) were mounted on glass slides and left to dry overnight at room temperature. Immediately thereafter the slides were incubated overnight with primary antibodies (pro-SP-C and Ki-67, diluted 1:400 and 1:25, respectively) or respective isotype IgG. Incubation with secondary antibodies (Alexa 555 anti-rabbit IgG and Alexa 488 anti-rat IgG) diluted in BSA 0.1%/PBS (1:1000) was performed for 1 h at room temperature, the slides were then washed, mounted with a DAPI-containing mounting medium and left to dry overnight. Slides were analysed with a Leica DM 2000 fluorescent microscope at the indicated magnification using Leica digital imaging software.

3.6.2. Flow cytometry

For flow cytometric antigen detection AEC grown on transwells were trypsinized (Trypsin/EDTA 1x, 1-2 min), pooled (3-5 transwells) and washed once in PBS. Subsequently AEC (cultured or freshly isolated) or lung homogenate samples were fixed for 15 min in 1% paraformaldehyde (PFA)/PBS solution (4° C), washed once in FACS buffer (PBS$^{-/-}$ supplemented with 7.4% (v/v) EDTA and 0.5% (v/v) FCS), and then incubated for 15 min in Saponin buffer (0.2% Saponin in FACS buffer) for permeabilization and hence detection of both, extracellular (CD45 and T1-α) and intracellular antigens (pro-SP-C, Ki-67). Unspecific antibody binding was inhibited by adding 10 μl Fc-Block. Subsequently, the cells were incubated with primary antibodies pro-SP-C (diluted 1:000), PE-conjugated Ki-67 (undiluted), biotinylated CD-45 (1:100) and T1-α (1:250), or with respective isotype IgG antibodies. The cells were then stained with the secondary antibodies (Alexa 488 or Alexa 647 anti-rabbit IgG and Alexa 647 or Alexa 488 anti-hamster IgG, all diluted 1:500 in Saponin buffer) for 20 min at 4°C. Immediately thereafter, where applicable, the cells were incubated with 5 μl streptavidin-conjugated APC-Cy7 antibody (1:100 diluted), for 3 min. Primary and secondary antibody excess was removed by two subsequent washes in Saponin buffer. Flow cytometry analysis was performed using a FACSCanto flow cytometer equipped with FACSDiva and WinMDI 2.8 software packages.

3.6.3. Western Blot

AEC were washed once with cold PBS (4° C) and lysed in 50 μl lysis buffer (see below). The cell lysate was incubated on ice for 15 min and immediately thereafter centrifuged at 13 000 rpm for 15 min at 4° C. The supernatant was separated from the cell pellet and protein content was determined by using a commercial spectrophotometric assay, Bio-Rad DC (detergent compatible). The assay is similar to the well-documented Lowry assay (85). Proteins (5-10 μg) were separated according to the size by SDS-polyacrylamide gel electrophoresis (SDS-PAGE) under reducing and denaturing conditions in 1 x SDS-running buffer (80 V, 40 mA, 2 h). Gels were composed of 5% stacking and 10% running gel. Prior to loading, proteins were mixed with loading buffer and boiled for 5 min on 95° C.

Materials and Methods

Lysis buffer

Tris (pH 7.5)	20 mM
NaCl	150 mM
Na_2EDTA	1 mM
EGTA	1 mM
NP-40	0.5 %
Na_3VO_4	2 mM
Protease inhibitor mix	1x (Roche)

1 x SDS running buffer

Tris	25 mM
Glycine	250 mM
SDS	0.1% (v/v)

Stacking gel (5%)

Tris (pH 6.8)	125 mM
Acrylamide	5 %
SDS	0.1% (v/v)
Temed	0.2% (v/v)
APS	0.05% (w/v)

Running gel (10%)

Tris (pH 8.8)	375 mM
Acrylamide	10 %
SDS	0.1% (v/v)
Temed	0.1% (v/v)
APS	0.03% (w/v)

Separated proteins from the gels were then transferred onto hybond-P PVDF-membrane using the Bio-Rad transfer chamber and transfer buffer, at 120 V and 265 mA, for 1 h. Membranes were then blocked for 30 min with a blocking buffer, and subsequently incubated overnight at 4°C with anti-STAT5 or anti-phospho STAT5 antibodies (both diluted 1:1000 in blocking buffer). After washing with washing buffer they were then incubated with 1:1000 diluted anti-rabbit horseradish peroxidase–conjugated secondary antibody. Final detection of protein was performed using the enhanced chemiluminescent Western blotting system and recorded on an autoradiograph. To remove bound antibodies and to reprobe the membranes, they were incubated at room temperature for 1 h in stripping buffer containing PBS/0.1 M glycine/0.375% HCl.

Transfer buffer (pH 7.4)	
Tris	25 mM
Glycine	192 mM
Methanol	20% (v/v)

Washing buffer	
PBS	1 x
dH$_2$O	
Tween 20	0.1 % (v/v)

Blocking buffer	
Non-fat dry milk	5% (w/v)
PBS	1 x
Tween 20	0.1 % (v/v)

Stripping buffer	
Glycine	0.1 M
dH$_2$O	
HCl	0.375%

3.6.4. Cytokine quantification

Cytokine levels in cell culture supernatants and bronchoalveolar lavage fluid were measured using commercially available sandwich ELISA kits. Standards, control, and samples were pipetted into the wells, incubated for 2 h at RT, followed by five washing steps with an ELISA autowasher. After 2 h of incubation with the conjugate solution and repetitive washing, substrate solution was added to each well for 30 min, and then the reaction was stopped. Optical density was measured using a microplate reader set to 450 nm; the sample values were read off the standard curve. Detection limits were 7.8 pg/ml for GM-CSF, 5.1 pg/ml for TNF-α, 2 pg/ml for CCL2 and 1.5 pg/ml for MIP-2.

3.7. *In vitro* proliferation assays

3.7.1. [^{3}H]-thymidine incorporation

Freshly isolated AEC II were maintained 16 h in medium supplemented with 10% FCS followed by 8-10 h of starvation (medium with 0.1% FCS) to achieve growth arrest before stimulation (recombinant TNF-α or GM-CSF) or begin of co-culture with AMφ, for 48 h. [^{3}H]-thymidine (0.25 µCi/well) was added in the culture wells for the final 5 h of the incubation. Afterwards, supernatants were aspirated and the cells were washed three times with PBS before lysis with 0.5 M NaOH. Before measurement cell-culture plates with lysis solution were shaken for 30 min at RT. The cellular [^{3}H]-thymidine content of each well or transwell was quantified by scintillation counting. In every experiment each condition was performed in quadruplicates. Results are expressed as fold induction of untreated cells (i.e. AEC in starving medium (0.1% FCS)).

3.7.2. Cell counting

For cell counting AEC were treated in the same way as for [^{3}H]-thymidine incorporation (*Section 3.7.1.*). After 48 and 72 h of stimulation, in mono/co-culture and matrigel:collagen mono/co-culture respectively, the cells were counted in a haemocytometer and by flow cytometry. Briefly, following trypsinization or matrigel:collagen release AEC were washed once in PBS and subsequently the cell pellet was resuspended in 120 µl of FACS buffer – 10 µl cell suspension were used for hemacytometer counting and 110 µl for flow-cytometry (60 sec, medium speed for each sample). The results are presented as fold induction of untreated AEC (in 0.1 % FCS).

3.8. *In vivo* mouse treatment protocols

Mice were sedated with xylazine hydrochloride (2.5 mg/kg, im) and ketamine hydrochloride (50 mg/kg, im), followed by fur/skin desinfection and subsequent shaving of the area above the trachea. A small incision was made and surrounding tissue bluntly dissected to expose the trachea. An Abbocath catheter was inserted in the trachea and subsequently LPS (10 µg/mouse) dissolved in sterile PBS in a total volume of 70 µl was slowly instilled, under stereomicroscopic control. Subsequently the skin was sutured; mice were left to recover from anaesthesia and then returned to their cages, with free access to food and water (3, 86). Wild type (wt), $GM^{-/-}$ and SPC-GM mice were intratracheally challenged with LPS for different time intervals (6, 12, 24, 48, 96, 148 and 240 h). In selected experiments LPS was applied together with function blocking anti-TNF-α antibodies or respective isotype IgG control antibodies (10 µg/mouse) for 6 or 96 h, in a total volume of 70 µl.

3.9. Collection and analysis of blood samples and bronchoalveolar lavage fluid (BALF)

Mice were sacrificed with an overdose of Isoflurane at the indicated time intervals, and the abdominal cavity was opened to expose the inferior vena cava. Blood was drawn with a 23-gauge cannula connected to a 1 ml syringe, and immediately thereafter transferred into a 1.5 ml collection tube.

The bronchoalveolar lavage fluid was collected as follows: the trachea was exposed and cannulated by a shortened 21-gauge cannula connected to a 1 ml syringe, followed by consecutive instillation and collection of 300, 400 and 500 µl of ice-cold 2 mM EDTA/PBS (concentrated BAL fluid). The cells from concentrated BALF were separated by centrifugation (1400 rpm, 10 min, 4° C), whereas the supernatant was harvested into a collection tube and was further used for cytokine quantification or alveolar leakage determination (see *Sections 3.6.4* and *3.10*). Subsequently, BAL was completed with additional instillation-collection cycles of 500 µl EDTA/PBS, until the final volume of 4 ml was recovered (diluted BAL fluid). After centrifugation (1400 rpm, 10 min, 4° C) the cells from diluted BALF samples were resuspended in 1 ml RPMI (supplemented with L-glutamine, 10% FCS and antibiotics) and pooled together with the cells from concentrated BAL. The supernatants from diluted BAL were discarded. The cell number in the pooled samples was counted in a haemocytometer, and was defined as total BALF leukocytes. BALF leukocyte subpopulations were determined by Pappenheim-stained cytocentrifuge preparations, as described in *Section 3.9.1*. For further flow cytometric analysis of BALF cells, the pooled samples were fixed in 1% PFA/PBS solution (15 min, on ice) and subsequently handled as described in *Section 3.6.2*.

3.9.1. Pappenheim-stained cytocentrifuge preparations

For identification and quantification of leukocyte subpopulations in pooled BAL samples Pappenheim staining of cytocentrifuge preparations were used (87). Briefly, cytospins were prepared from every pooled BALF sample, containing 30000-50000 cells in 100 µl, and subsequently stained for 5 min in May-Grünwald stain and 10 min in 5% of Giemsa Azur-Eosin-Methylenblue solution. Total resident alveolar macrophages and neutrophil numbers in BALF were determined by differential cell counts using overall morphological criteria, including differences in cells size and shape of nuclei, and subsequent multiplication of obtained percentage values with the respective total BALF leukocyte counts.

3.10. *In vivo* lung permeability assay

For the determination of alveolar leakage mice received an intravenous injection (into the tail vein) of 1 mg FITC-labelled albumin in 100 µl of sterile NaCl 0.9%. 45 min later, BALF and blood samples were collected as described in *Section 3.9*. Blood samples were incubated for 3 h at RT until coagulation occurred and serum was recovered after centrifugation (4000 rpm, 15 min, RT). FITC fluorescence was measured in duplicates in concentrated BAL fluid and serum samples (diluted 1:100 in PBS) and compared to standard samples serially diluted 1:10 with PBS, using a fluorescence spectrophotometer operating at 488 nm absorbance and 525 ± 20 nm emission wavelengths, respectively. The lung permeability index is defined as the ratio of fluorescence signals of concentrated BALF samples to fluorescence signals of 1:100 diluted serum samples and given as arbitrary units (AU).

3.11. Measurement of *in vivo* proliferation of AEC II

The proportion of proliferating AEC II in lung homogenates was investigated by flow cytometric staining with antibodies detecting the proliferation marker Ki-67. Lung homogenate samples were prepared as described in *Section 3.2.*, the cells were fixed and permeabilized (*Section 3.6.2.*) and subsequently co-stained with Ki-67 PE-conjugated antibody, pro-SP-C and CD45 antibodies. Proliferating AEC II were determined as the Ki-67$^+$ sub-population from CD45$^-$/pro-SP-C$^+$ cells, analysed against an isotype IgG control.

3.11.1. Total AEC numbers in lung homogenates

Total numbers of AEC II and AEC I in lung homogenates were determined by multiplying the percentage of pro-SP-C$^+$ and T1-α^+ cells, respectively (defined by flow cytometric staining) with the total lung homogenate cell counts (obtained with hemacytometer). Subsequently, total AEC numbers were calculated as a sum of total AEC II and AEC I numbers.

3.12. Infection experiments with *K. pneumoniae*

The *K. pneumoniae* serotype 2 strain was purchased from ATCC (No 43816). *K. pneumoniae* was grown in Todd-Hewitt broth for 18-24 h. Determination of colony-forming units (CFU) was done by plating tenfold serial dilutions of bacterial suspensions on McConkey agar plates followed by incubation of the plates at 37°C for 18 hours and enumeration of the CFU. Bacteria were then diluted with PBS to the desired concentration (25 x 10^4 CFU/70 µl per mouse) and used for intratracheal infection. The procedure was in analogy to the intratracheal application of LPS (see section 3.8).

4. Results

4.1. LPS-stimulation of AMφ induces AEC growth factors in co-culture

Keratinocyte growth factor (KGF), vascular endothelial growth factor (VEGF), platelet – derived growth factor (PDGF) and granulocyte macrophage colony-stimulating factor (GM-CSF) have all been described as potent epithelial mitogens (60, 75, 88-91). To investigate whether AMφ are capable to induce expression of these growth factors in alveolar epithelial cells under inflammatory conditions, AEC were either mono- or co-cultured with AMφ for 48 h, and treated with LPS (1 µg/ml for 48 h) or left untreated. Analysis of gene expression of the aforementioned growth factors in AEC revealed a significant upregulation of KGF, VEGF, PDGFa and, most prominent, of GM-CSF mRNA in AEC co-cultured with LPS-stimulated AMφ compared to AEC in monoculture. Of note, LPS stimulation of mono-cultured AEC or unstimulated AEC/AMφ co-culture revealed no significant upregulation of any of the analysed growth factors in AEC (Fig. 5A). In contrast to the findings in AEC, AMφ did not show any significant regulation of the gene products named above, nor did co-culture with AEC influence their expression irrespective of the absence or presence of LPS (Fig. 5B). Additionally, expression of several other growth factors in AEC was analysed (Table 1), but only non-significant changes were observed upon LPS stimulation and co-culture with LPS-stimulated AMφ. Hence, a slight upregulation of fibroblast growth factor 2 (FGF2) and platelet derived growth factor b (PDGFb) and downregulation of platelet derived growth factor d (PDGFd) were noted in AEC co-cultured with LPS-stimulated AMφ.

Given that, among the growth factors analysed, GM-CSF mRNA upregulation was most pronounced, GM-CSF protein release in mono- and co-culture upon LPS stimulation was further investigated. As demonstrated in Fig. 6, AMφ alone did not release significant amounts of GM-CSF into the supernatant, irrespectively of the presence or absence of LPS. AEC alone showed remarkably higher release of GM-CSF compared to AMφ, which was not significantly enhanced in presence of LPS. Supernatants from LPS-stimulated co-cultures, however, contained significantly higher amounts of GM-CSF than supernatants from AEC mono-cultures or from unstimulated co-cultures. Of note, presence of AMφ reduced GM-CSF levels observed in AEC mono-culture (Fig. 6, lanes 3-5), most likely due to macrophage GM-CSF consumption. Collectively, these data indicate that AEC are the primary alveolar source of epithelial growth factors and that AMφ have the potential to significantly amplify epithelial expression of various growth factors, in particular of epithelial GM-CSF, upon inflammatory stimulation.

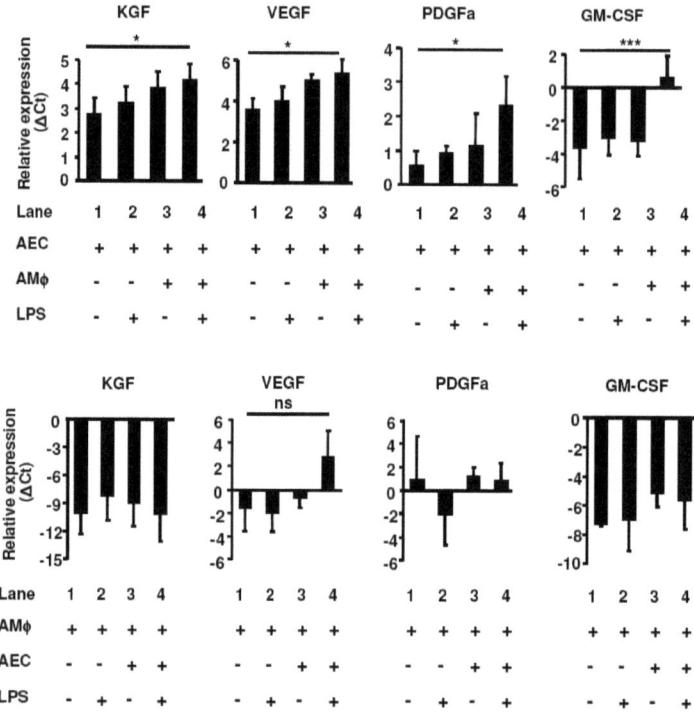

Figure 5. LPS-stimulated AMφ enhance the expression of growth factors in co-cultured AEC. Freshly isolated AEC cultured for 60 h on transwells were either mono-cultured and left unstimulated or were stimulated with LPS (1 µg/ml), or were co-cultured with unstimulated or LPS-stimulated resident AMφ for 48 h. Subsequently, relative gene expression of different growth factors was analysed in both cell types. (A) Relative mRNA expression of KGF, VEGF, PDGFa and GM-CSF, in unstimulated or LPS-treated mono-cultured AEC (lanes 1 and 2) or co-cultured AEC (lanes 3 and 4). (B) Relative mRNA expression of KGF, VEGF, PDGFa, and GM-CSF in unstimulated or LPS-treated mono-cultured AMφ (lanes 1 and 2) or co-cultured AMφ (lanes 3 and 4). Values are means ± SD from at least n=3 different experiments each of which was performed in triplicates; *p<0.05, ***p<0.001. ns, not significant.

Results

Gene symbol	Gene name	Relative gene expression (ΔCt)			
		AEC	AEC + LPS	AEC (AMφ)	AEC (AMφ + LPS)
IGF-1	Insulin-like growth factor 1	3.6±0.5	3.8± 0.2	4.1±0.5	3.2±0.5
IGF-2	Insulin-like growth factor 2	-2.4± 0.7	-2.63±1.0	-1.9±0.2	-2.9±1.5
TGFα	Transforming growth factor-alpha	-2.9±0.6	-3.2±0.5	-4.0±0.3	-3.7±0.1
FGF2	Fibroblast growth factor 2	1.9±0.4	1.9±0.7	2.1±0.3	2.7±0.9
PDGFb	Platelet derived growth factor – b	-6.9±2.7	-6.4±0.6	-7.1±0.4	-5.1±1.1
PDGFc	Platelet derived growth factor – c	-1.4± 0.7	-1.5± 0.0	-1.1±0.0	0.3± 0.9
PDGFd	Platelet derived growth factor – d	-0.7±0.7	-0.1±0.6	-1.8±0.5	-2.5±0.3

Table 1. mRNA expression of growth factors in AEC mono or co-cultured, in the presence or absence of LPS.

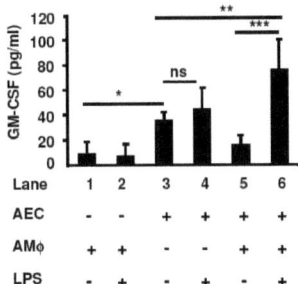

Figure 6. GM-CSF secretion in the supernatants from AEC/AMφ co-culture. GM-CSF release from mono-cultured AMφ (lanes 1 and 2), mono-cultured AEC (lanes 3 and 4) and AEC/AMφ co-cultures (lanes 5 and 6) in the presence or absence of LPS was analysed by ELISA. All given values are means ± SD from n=5 different experiments each of which was performed in triplicates; *p<0.05, **p<0.01, ***p<0.001; ns, non-significant.

4.2. Epithelial GM-CSF expression is induced by alveolar macrophage TNF-α

Given that LPS-stimulated AMφ induced GM-CSF expression in AEC, most likely by a soluble mediator, it was further assumed that the pro-inflammatory TNF-α might mediate these effects. AMφ secrete significant amounts of the pro-inflammatory cytokine TNF-α upon LPS treatment and in early phase of gram-negative infections (92, 93), and AEC are known to respond to TNF-α (43, 94). Accordingly, TNF-α solely originated from AMφ in the LPS-treated AEC/AMφ co-cultures, whereas AEC did not release any detectable levels of TNF-α (Fig. 7, lanes 2 and 6).

Results

Of note, both TNF-α receptors 1 and 2 (TNFR1/2) were expressed on cultured AEC on mRNA level (Fig. 8).

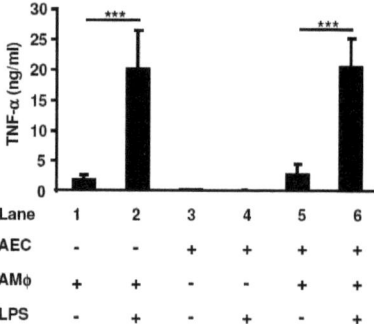

Figure 7. Quantification of TNF-α levels in AEC/AMφ co-culture. TNF-α levels in supernatants taken from unstimulated and LPS-stimulated mono- and co-cultured AEC and AMφ were determined by ELISA. All given values are presented as means ± SD from n=3 independent experiments. ***p<0.001.

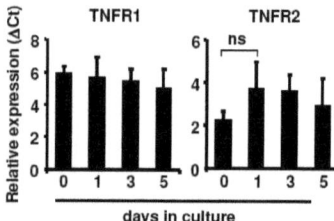

Figure 8. Expression of TNF-α receptors during AEC *in vitro* culture. Freshly isolated AEC were cultured for 5 days and mRNA expression of TNFR1 and TNFR2 was analysed at the indicated time-points. All values are presented as means ± SD from n=3 independent experiments. TNFR1, TNF-α receptor 1; TNFR2, TNF-α receptor 2.

To evaluate whether macrophage TNF-α induced GM-CSF production in AEC, neutralizing anti-TNF-α antibodies were applied in the co-culture model. Indeed, anti-TNF-α treatment significantly decreased epithelial GM-CSF expression in LPS-treated co-cultures, both on mRNA and protein level (Fig. 9).

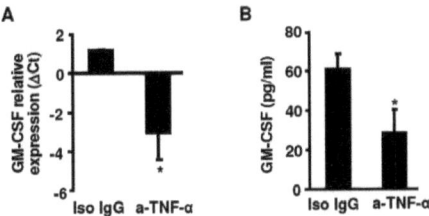

Figure 9. Alveolar macrophage TNF-α mediates epithelial GM-CSF production. Anti-TNF-α or isotype IgG antibodies were added to the medium of LPS-stimulated AEC/AMφ co-cultures (1 µg/ml at 2, 12 and 20 h post LPS treatment), and after 48 h GM-CSF mRNA expression in AEC (A) and GM-CSF protein in AEC/AMφ co-culture supernatants (B) were determined. All values are means ± SD from n=3 independent experiments. *p<0.05, a-TNF-α, anti-TNF-α antibody; Iso IgG, isotype IgG.

Moreover, stimulation of mono-cultured AEC with recombinant murine TNF-α resulted in increased expression of GM-CSF, both on mRNA and protein level in a time-dependent manner. The highest GM-CSF levels were observed at 48 h of TNF-α stimulation (Fig. 10). Taken together, these data demonstrate that macrophage TNF-α, released upon LPS recognition, induces GM-CSF expression in co-cultured AEC, indicating that resident lung macrophages induce the release of epithelial growth factors from AEC yet in the early phase of inflammation.

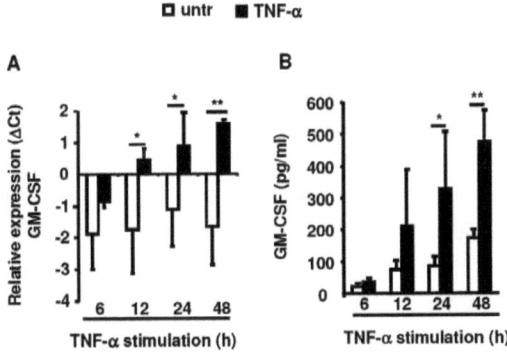

Figure 10. Recombinant TNF-α induces GM-CSF production in AEC *in vitro*. AEC were stimulated with 100 ng/ml recombinant murine TNF-α for 6, 12, 24 and 48 h, and subsequently relative GM-CSF mRNA expression (A) and GM-CSF protein levels in culture supernatants (B) were measured. Values are means ± SD from n=3 independent experiments. *p<0.05, **p<0.01. Untr, untreated.

4.3. GM-CSF receptor expression is associated with the AEC II phenotype

To evaluate the GM-CSF signalling in epithelial cells, initially the expression of both GM-CSF receptor subunits (α and ß) over the 5 days of *in vitro* culture was investigated. As shown in Fig. 11, freshly isolated AEC expressed both subunits of the GM-CSF receptor, but their expression decreased during 5 days of culture.

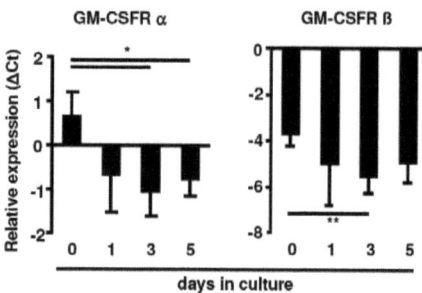

Figure 11. Freshly isolated AEC express both GM-CSF receptor subunits. GM-CSF receptor (α and ß) relative expression was determined over 5 days of *in vitro* culture. Values are means ± SD from n=4 independent experiments. *p<0.05, **p<0.01. GM-CSFRα, GM-CSF receptor alpha subunit; GM-CSFRß, GM-CSF receptor beta subunit.

Given that rat and human AEC II cultured on plastic cell-culture plates have been shown to change their phenotype during *in vitro* culture, acquiring features of AEC I (15, 95), it was further examined whether GMCSF receptor subunit expression might be related to the AEC II phenotype. Indeed, mRNA expression of the AEC II specific markers such as pro-SP-C (5), CCAAT enhancer binding protein alpha (C/EBPα) (96) and gamma amino-butyric acid pi-subunit (GABRP) (97) was pronounced at day 0, and rapidly declined during 5 days of culture, whereas mRNA levels of the AEC I marker T1-α increased (98) (Fig. 12A).

In addition, immunolabelling of these markers revealed corresponding results on protein level, as demonstrated by flow cytometry (representative dot plots, Fig. 12B and quantitative analyses of the respective proportions of pro-SP-C$^+$ or T1-α$^+$ AEC, Fig. 12C) and immunofluorescence (Fig. 12D). Of note, GM-CSF stimulation of AEC (Fig. 12A) did not influence AEC phenotype changes.

Together, these data indicate that GM-CSF receptor subunits α and ß are expressed on freshly isolated AEC. Thus, epithelial expression of GM-CSF receptors is associated with the AEC type II phenotype, and decreased with *in vitro* trans-differentiation into AEC I-like cells.

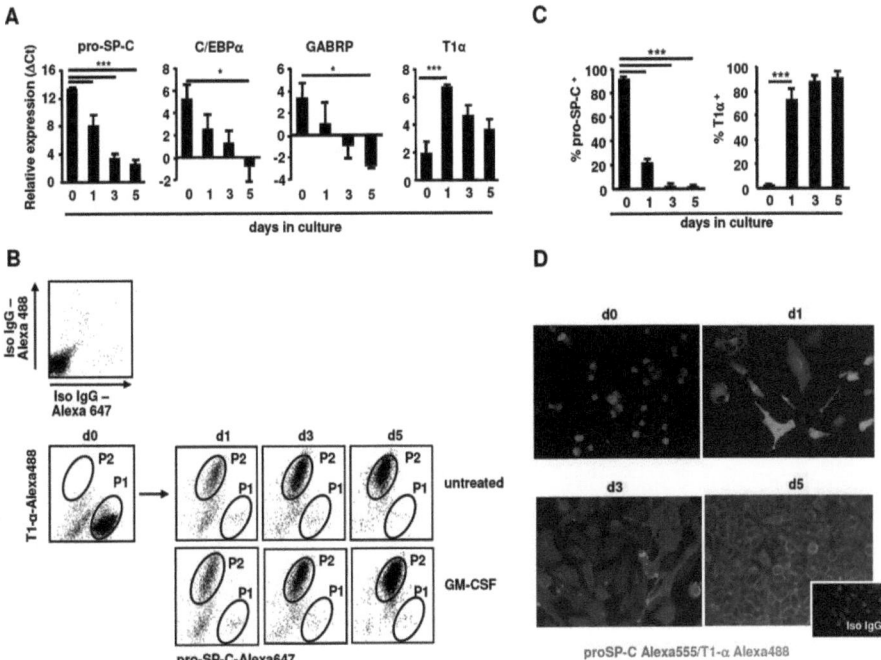

Figure 12. Expression changes of the markers of type II and type I AEC phenotype during 5 days of culture of untreated or GM-CSF-treated AEC. (A) Relative expression of AEC II (pro SP-C, C/EBPα and GABRP) and AEC I (T1-α) markers. (B) Representative dot plots of pro-SP-C and T1-α expression of AEC at d 0, 1, 3, and 5 post isolation, untreated or GM-CSF stimulated, including staining with respective isotype controls. (C) Bar diagram representing the percentages of pro-SP-C$^+$ (P1) and T1-α$^+$ (P2) cells as gated in B. Values are presented as means ± SD from 3 independent experiments. (D) Representative immmunofluorescence staining of AEC at day 0, 1, 3 and 5 with pro-SP-C (red) and T1-α (green), or respective isotype IgG; magnification x20. *p<0.05, ***p<0.001. Iso IgG, isotype IgG control.

Results

4.4. GM-CSF signalling in AEC

4.4.1. GM-CSF stimulation is not associated with pro-inflammatory cytokine production in AEC

Tanimoto *et al.* have recently demonstrated that GM-CSF stimulates pro-inflammatory cytokine production, such as monocyte chemoattractant protein-/CC-chemokine ligand 2 (CCL2), via induction of the STAT5/JAK2 pathway (99). To investigate whether epithelial cells may respond in a similar manner to GM-CSF, AEC were stimulated at day 1 of culture with GM-CSF for various time intervals, and measured release of the major monocyte and neutrophil chemoattractants, CCL2 and MIP-2 (macrophage inflammatory protein 2) by ELISA. As demonstrated in Fig. 13, GM-CSF did not induce production of the chemokines CCL2 and MIP-2 in AEC, indicating that GM-CSF did not initiate a pro-inflammatory response in AEC.

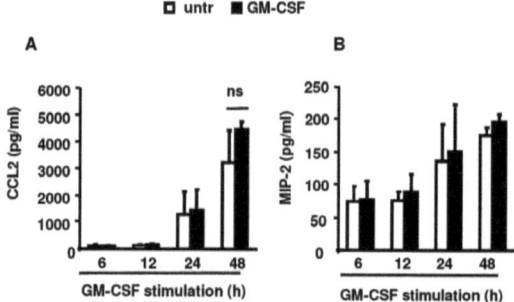

Figure 13. GM-CSF does not induce the release of pro-inflammatory chemokines in AEC. AEC at day 1 of culture were stimulated with 100 ng/ml GM-CSF for 6, 12, 24 and 48 h and subsequently CCL2 (A) and MIP-2 (B) production was determined in supernatants by ELISA. Untreated AEC were used as a control at each time point. Values are means ± SD from n=3 independent experiments. untr, untreated; ns, not significant.

4.4.2. AEC do not produce growth factors upon GM-CSF treatment

Huffman Reed *et al* (75) suggested that the observed AEC II hyperplasia in the lungs of SPC-GM may be indirectly mediated by GM-CSF-dependent induction of potent epithelial growth factors in epithelial cells. To evaluate this hypothesis AEC were stimulated at day 1 of culture with GM-CSF for 24 h and subsequently mRNA expression of several epithelial growth factors was analysed. However, non significant differences between untreated and GM-CSF stimulated AEC were observed, indicating that GM-CSF does not enhance expression of further epithelial growth factors in AEC (Table 2).

Results

Gene symbol	Gene name	Relative gene expression (ΔCt)	
		untreated	GM-CSF
IGF-1	Insulin-like growth factor 1	-1.26±0.7	-1.8±0.1
IGF-2	Insulin-like growth factor 2	-2.0± 1.1	-2.6±0.5
TGFα	Transforming growth factor-alpha	-0.8±0.4	-0.9±1.4
FGF2	Fibroblast growth factor 2	0.4±0.8	-0.1±0.6
PDGFa	Platelet derived growth factor – a	0.8±0.6	0.2±0.6
PDGFb	Platelet derived growth factor – b	-5.7± 1.5	-6.4± 2.0
PDGFc	Platelet derived growth factor – c	-1.0±0.7	-1.6±0.7
PDGFd	Platelet derived growth factor – d	-4.0±2.0	-5.4±0.6
VEGF	Vascular endothelial growth factor	3.0±1.4	3.2±1.4
KGF	Keratinocyte growth factor	1.8±1.0	2.4±0.9

Table 2. Relative expression of growth factors in AEC after GM-CSF stimulation for 24 h at day 1 of AEC culture.

4.4.3. GM-CSF induces proliferative signalling in AEC

GM-CSF receptor downstream signalling has been described to be mediated by various intracellular pathways involving STATs, MAPK and PI3K/Akt (100, 101). Stimulation of AEC at day 1 of culture with recombinant murine GM-CSF, induced rapid and transient phosphorylation of STAT5 (Fig. 14). STAT5 phosphorylation revealed to be associated with increased mRNA expression of the proliferation marker Cyclin D1 after 24 h of stimulation (Fig.15).

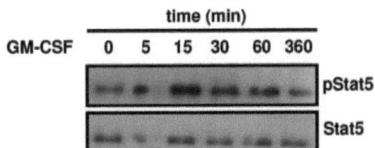

Figure 14. GM-CSF induces STAT5 phosphorylation in AEC. Representative western blot analysis of STAT5 phosphorylation in AEC stimulated with GM-CSF (500 pg/ml) at day 1 of culture for the indicated time points, total STAT5 was used as a loading control.

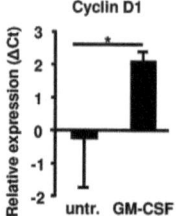

Figure 15. Cyclin D1 mRNA expression is upregulated upon GM-CSF stimulation of AEC. AEC at day 1 of culture were stimulated with GM-CSF (100 ng/ml) for 24 h, and subsequently Cyclin D1 mRNA expression was analysed. Untreated AEC were used as a control. Values are means ± SD from n=3 independent experiments. *p<0.05; untr, untreated.

Moreover, GM-CSF stimulation of AEC at day 1, but not at day 3 of culture, resulted in increased proliferation, as assessed by [^{3}H]-thymidine incorporation and cell-counting (Fig. 16). Collectively, these data indicate that a STAT5-dependent intracellular signal is induced upon GM-CSF receptor binding in day 1 AEC, resulting in Cyclin D1 expression and most likely mediating the subsequent proliferation.

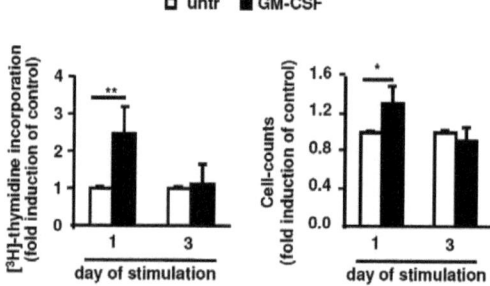

Figure 16. GM-CSF induces increased AEC proliferation. Freshly isolated AEC were left to adhere for 16 h, were then serum starved for 10 h and immediately thereafter stimulated with GM-CSF for 48 h. Likewise, AEC at day 3 of culture were stimulated with GM-CSF for 48 h in serum starving medium. Subsequently, AEC proliferation was measured by [^{3}H]-thymidine incorporation (A) and cell counting (B). Data is presented as fold induction of untreated control; values are means ± SD from n=4 independent experiments performed in quadruplicate for [^{3}H]-thymidine incorporation, and n=3 for cell-counting. *p<0.05, **p<0.01. Untr, untreated.

Of note, day 1 AEC, despite acquisition of the type I phenotype in terms of marker expression, were still capable to respond to the proliferative GM-CSF signal as opposed to day 3 AEC, indicating that day 1 AEC might functionally still possess type II characteristics during transition towards the type I phenotype. Likewise, AEC grown on matrigel:collagen matrix, thereby maintained in the "classical" type II phenotype until day 3 of culture (Fig. 17), similarly expressed and released GM-CSF upon LPS stimulation in the co-culture and responded to GM-CSF stimulation with enhanced proliferation (Fig. 18), further supporting the concept that the proliferative response to GM-CSF is related to the type II AEC phenotype.

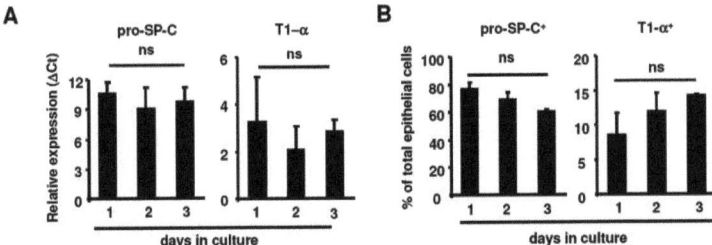

Figure 17. Matrigel:collagen culture delays *in vitro* differentiation of murine AEC. Freshly isolated AEC were seeded on matrigel:collagen pre-coated wells of 24-well plate and cultured for up to 3 days. (A) Relative mRNA expression of pro-SP-C and T1-α in AEC analysed at day 1, 2 and 3 of culture. (B) Flow cytometry quantification of pro-SP-C$^+$ and T1-α$^+$ cells; bar graphs show cells percentage of total epithelial cells. Values are presented as means ± SD from 3 independent experiments. ns, non-significant.

Results

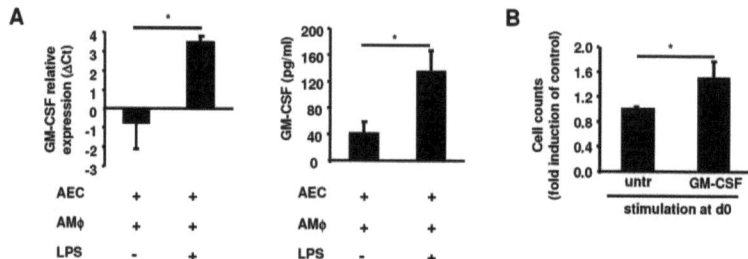

Figure 18. Matrigel:collagen cultured AEC express GM-CSF in co-culture with LPS stimulated AMφ and proliferate upon GM-CSF stimulation. Following isolation, AEC were left to attach for 5 h on matrigel:collagen mixture, and immediately thereafter either co-cultured with unstimulated or LPS-stimulated AMφ or treated with GM-CSF. (A) After 48 h of co-culture AEC were released from the gel and GM-CSF relative mRNA expression (left diagram) and protein secretion into the co-culture supernatants (right diagram) were determined. Values are presented as means ± SD from 3 independent experiments. (B) After 72 h of GM-CSF stimulation AEC proliferation was assessed by cell counting. Data is presented as fold induction of untreated control; values are means ± SD from 3 independent experiments; *p<0.05; untr, untreated.

4.5. AEC proliferation is induced by macrophage TNF-α and mediated by GM-CSF

Given that GM-CSF induced proliferative signalling in AEC at day 1 of culture and macrophage TNF-α stimulated GM-CSF expression in epithelial cells, the hypothesis that AEC proliferation might be induced by TNF-α in a GM-CSF dependent manner was tested. Therefore, AEC isolated from GM-CSF-deficient mice ($GM^{-/-}$ AEC) were stimulated at day 1 of culture with recombinant TNF-α and compared with wild type AEC (wt AEC) for proliferation, assessed by [^{3}H]-thymidine incorporation and cell counting. As given in Fig. 19A, $GM^{-/-}$ AEC did not show enhanced proliferation upon TNF-α stimulation, whereas TNF-α stimulated wt AEC demonstrated significantly increased proliferation, compared to untreated control (*grey bars*).

Similarly, to evaluate whether LPS-stimulated AMφ may induce proliferation of epithelial cells via GM-CSF, $GM^{-/-}$ AEC grown on transwells were co-cultured with wt AMφ, with or without LPS and compared to co-cultured wt AEC for proliferation. Interestingly, wt AEC co-cultured with AMφ in the presence of LPS showed remarkably increased [^{3}H]-thymidine incorporation and AEC counts compared to unstimulated wt AEC in mono-culture, whereas LPS-stimulated AMφ did not influence the proliferation of $GM^{-/-}$ AEC (*black bars*). Likewise,

LPS-stimulated AMφ induced increased cell counts of the co-cultured wt AEC grown on matrigel:collagen matrix (i.e. "classical" AEC II), as shown on Fig. 19B.

Collectively, this data clearly demonstrate that macrophage TNF-α released upon LPS stimulation, induces GM-CSF secretion in AEC which in turn induces AEC proliferation by an autocrine stimulation loop *in vitro*.

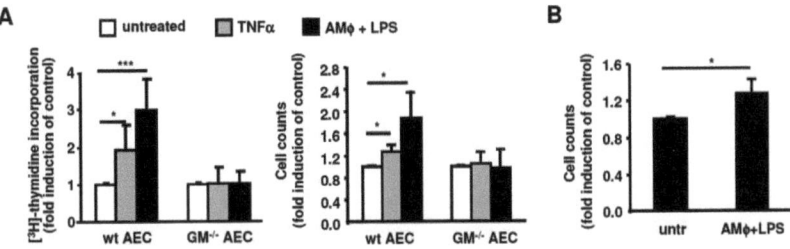

Figure 19. GM-CSF mediates macrophage TNF-α induced AEC proliferation. (A) AEC monocultures from wt and GM$^{-/-}$ mice were stimulated with recombinant TNF-α (100 ng/ml) for 48 h (*grey bars*) and proliferation was assayed by [^{3}H]-thymidine incorporation (*left panel*) and cell counting (*right panel*). For proliferation analysis of co-cultured epithelial cells, wt AEC or GM$^{-/-}$ AEC were plated on transwells and co-cultured with LPS-stimulated resident AMφ for 48 h before proliferation analysis (*black bars*). Data is presented as fold induction of untreated cells (*white bars*). (B) Freshly isolated AEC were cultured on matrigel:collagen matrix, left to attach for 5 h and immediately thereafter co-cultured with LPS-stimulated AMφ. Cell counts were determined after 72 h of co-culture. Values are means ± SD from at least n=4 independent experiments performed in quadruplicates (for [^{3}H]-thymidine incorporation) and n=3 for cell counting. *$p<0.05$, ***$p<0.001$; wt, wild type; untr, untreated.

4.6. TNF-α mediates AEC II proliferation following LPS-induced lung injury *in vivo*

To evaluate the potential of macrophage TNF-α to mediate AEC II proliferation in LPS-induced acute lung injury *in vivo*, AEC II proliferation at 96 h post LPS instillation was analysed in wt mice treated intratracheally with either anti-TNF-α or isotype control antibodies. Proliferating AEC II in lung homogenate samples were defined as CD45$^-$/pro-SP-C$^+$/Ki67$^+$, as demonstrated in the representative FACS plots in Fig. 20A. A remarkable increase in the percentage of proliferating AEC II was observed in LPS-injured mice after 4 days post LPS installation compared to untreated mice. Interestingly, anti-TNF-α treatment significantly reduced the proliferating proportion of AEC II in LPS-challenged wt mice compared to treatment with isotype control antibodies (Fig. 20B). This finding was additionally supported by immunofluorescence analysis of whole lung tissue slices co-stained for pro-SP-C and Ki-67, demonstrating that anti-TNF-α treatment markedly reduces the proportion of proliferating AEC II after LPS-challenge (pro-SP-C$^+$/Ki-67$^+$ cells, Fig. 20C). Significant changes in the total AEC II numbers during the treatment were not observed (Fig. 20 D).

Analysis of GM-CSF levels in the BAL fluid after 6 h of LPS-induced lung injury in mice revealed significantly lower GM-CSF release from alveolar cells when mice were treated with anti-TNF-α antibodies as compared to isotype-treated mice (Fig. 21).

These data provide evidence that indeed macrophage TNF-α mediates alveolar epithelial cell proliferation *in vivo* following LPS-induced lung injury via induction of GM-CSF.

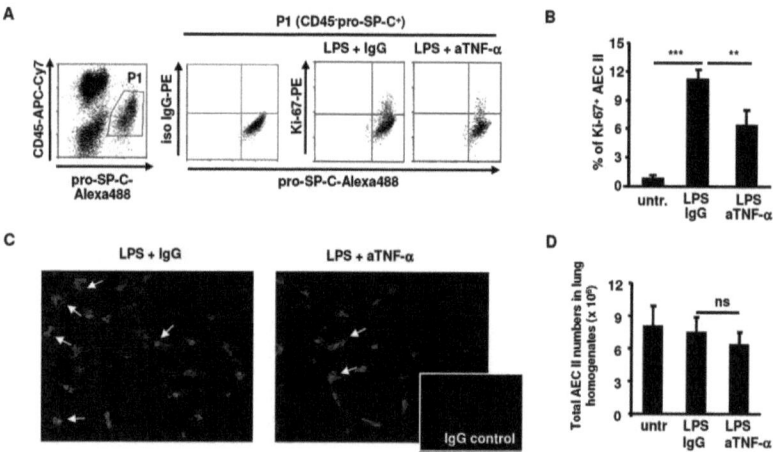

Figure 20. TNF-α mediates AEC II proliferation *in vivo*. (A) Flow cytometric analysis of AEC II proliferation following LPS-induced lung injury. Lung homogenates from wt mice treated intratracheally with 10 µg LPS plus either anti-TNF-α, or isotype IgG antibodies, respectively, were analysed for CD45, pro-SP-C and Ki-67 expression. Representative dot plots show co-expression of pro-SP-C and Ki-67 (or respective iso IgG) of CD45$^-$/pro-SP-C$^+$cells (P1). (B) Quantification of FACS analysis of proliferating AEC II; bar graphs show the percentage of Ki-67$^+$ of total AEC II (pro-SP-C$^+$/CD45$^-$) in lung homogenates. Values are means ± SD from n=3 mice per group. (C) Representative immunofluorescent staining of pro-SP-C (red) and Ki-67 (green), or respective IgG, performed on lung cryosections from wt mice treated with either LPS + IgG or LPS + anti-TNFα antibodies for 96 h. Arrows depict proliferating AEC II; magnification x 20. D) Total AEC II numbers in lung homogenates of untreated, LPS + IgG and LPS + aTNF-α treated mice. The graph represents total AEC II numbers obtained from the respective AEC II percentages and total cell numbers of homogenates. Values are means ± SD from n=3 mice per group. **p<0.01, ***p<0.001. aTNF-α, anti-TNF-α antibodies; IgG, isotype IgG antibodies; ns, non significant.

Results

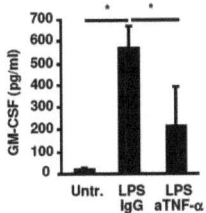

Figure 21. Neutralization of alveolar TNF-α reduces alveolar GM-CSF release after LPS challenge. Analysis of GM-CSF levels after 6 h of LPS in BALF from the various treatment groups was performed by ELISA. Values are means ± SD from n= 3 mice per group; *p<0.05. aTNF-α, anti-TNF-α antibodies; IgG, isotype IgG antibodies; untr, untreated.

4.7. GM-CSF enhances AEC II proliferation and alveolar barrier renewal after LPS-induced acute lung injury

To analyse the influence of GM-CSF on alveolar repair after LPS-induced lung injury *in vivo*, three groups of mice (wt, $GM^{-/-}$ and SPC-GM mice) were treated intratracheally with LPS for various time points and subjected to BAL for evaluation of amount and composition of alveolar leukocyte infiltration. As shown in Fig. 22, a pronounced accumulation of leukocytes was observed in the alveolar air spaces of all treatment groups between 12 and 48 h post LPS treatment.

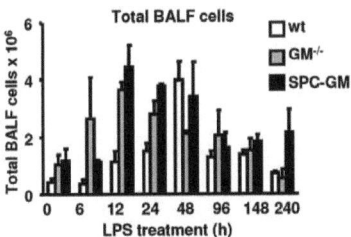

Figure 22. Quantification of total leukocyte numbers in BALF in wt (white bars), $GM^{-/-}$ (grey bars) and SPC-GM (black bars) mice in the time course post LPS instillation (n=3-5 mice per group, values are given as means ± SD).

Morphologic analysis of leukocyte subpopulations from Pappenheim-stainied BALF cytospin preparations revealed that accumulating alveolar leukocytes were predominantly neutrophils

(Fig. 23). Alveolar neutrophil peaks reached in wt, $GM^{-/-}$ and SPC-GM mice, were virtually identical.

$GM^{-/-}$ mice had similar resident AMφ counts as wt mice in the early stages of LPS-induced inflammation, but substantially lower AMφ numbers during the later stages (48 h to 240 h). Total BALF AMφ numbers were significantly higher in untreated SPC-GM mice as well as at all time intervals following LPS treatment compared to wt mice, an observation which has been described before (75, 77).

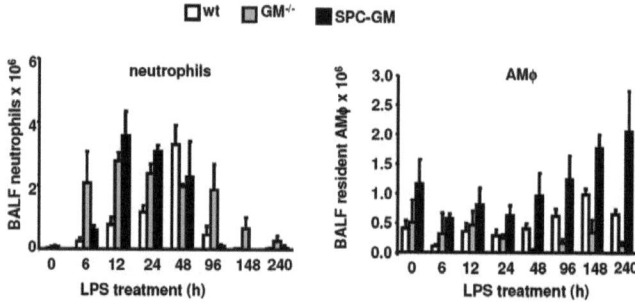

Figure 23. Quantification of BALF leukocyte subpopulations from Pappenheim-stained cytocentrifuged preparations. Data is given as total cells and represents means ± SD from n=3 animals per group; wt (white bars), $GM^{-/-}$ (grey bars) and SPC-GM (black bars).

Analysis of BALF TNF-α levels upon intratracheal LPS administration in the three different treatment groups demonstrated that TNF-α was alveolarly released in wt, $GM^{-/-}$ and SPC-GM mice, most prominent at 6 h (Fig. 24). GM-CSF was released into the alveolar space of wt mice at 6 h post LPS treatment and was undetectable in $GM^{-/-}$ mice. SPC-GM mice produced significantly higher amounts of GM-CSF at baseline conditions (0 h) and at 6 and 12 h post LPS treatment compared to wt mice (Fig. 24). Of note, GM-CSF levels in constitutively overexpressing SPC-GM mice decreased between 12 and 24 h post LPS administration, most likely due to consumption by alveolar neutrophils and macrophages.

Results

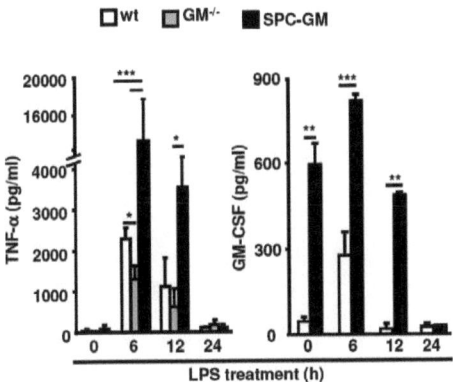

Figure 24. TNF-α and GM-CSF levels in BAL fluid from LPS-treated mice. Cytokine levels in BAL fluid of wt (white bars), GM$^{-/-}$ (grey bars) and SPC-GM (black bars) mice were quantified by ELISA; data is presented as means ± SD from n=3 mice per group; *p<0.05, **p<0.01, ***p<0.001.

To investigate the role of GM-CSF in alveolar epithelial repair processes following LPS-induced acute lung injury, AEC II proliferation in the various treatment groups was determined by flow cytometry and immunofluorescence on lung cryosections after 96 h post LPS instillation, a time point where recruited inflammatory leukocytes were virtually resolved from the air spaces and alveolar repair processes should likewise be initiated. As shown in Fig. 25A and B, proliferation of AEC type II was significantly higher in LPS-treated compared to untreated wt mice. Of note, the proliferating proportion of type II AEC was lower in GM$^{-/-}$ mice at 96 h post LPS administration, whereas in SPC-GM mice proliferation was comparable to wt mice. Likewise, the AEC II proportion in lung homogenates was significantly decreased in GM$^{-/-}$ mice and increased in SPC-GM mice compared to wt mice after 96 h post LPS instillation (Fig. 26A). In contrast, the percentage of AEC I (T1-α^{+} AEC) in lung homogenates was virtually identical before and after 96 h of LPS in all of the treatment groups (Fig. 26B). Similarly to AEC II proportions, the total AEC numbers (AEC II + AEC I) in GM$^{-/-}$ mice significantly declined following LPS treatment (Fig. 26C), indicating that the observed decrease in the AEC II percentages at the indicated time point (Fig. 24 A) is most likely due to LPS-mediated AEC II injury. Collectively, these findings suggest that epithelial GM-CSF induces AEC type II proliferation and that the lack of epithelial GM-CSF is associated with impaired AEC II renewal in LPS-induced lung injury.

49

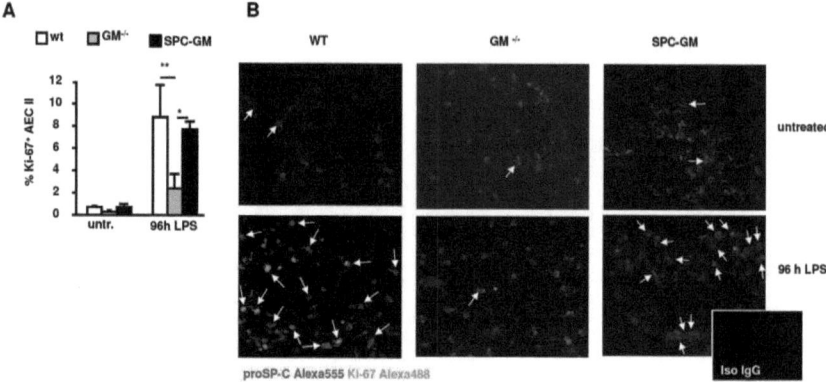

Figure 25. GM-CSF-deficiency is associated with decreased AEC II proliferation after LPS-induced lung injury. (A) Flow cytometric quantification of the proliferating proportion of AEC II in LPS-treated wt (white bars), GM$^{-/-}$ (grey bars) and SPC-GM (black bars). Bar graphs represent the percentage of Ki-67$^+$ of total AEC II (CD45$^-$/pro-SP-C$^+$) in lung homogenates from n=3 mice per group. Values are given as means ± SD. (B) Representative immunofluorescence staining of lung cryosections obtained from untreated or 96 h LPS-treated wt, GM$^{-/-}$ and SPC-GM mice. Arrows depict pro-SP-C (red) positive cells expressing Ki-67 (green); magnification x20; Iso IgG, isotype IgG control; untr, untreated. *p<0.05, **p<0.01.

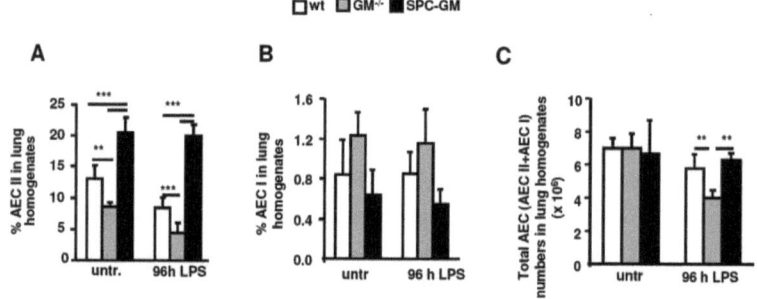

Figure 26. Reduction of total AEC numbers after LPS-induced lung injury is due to loss of AEC II but not of AEC I. The proportions and total AEC numbers in lung homogenates of untreated and LPS-treated wt (white bars), GM$^{-/-}$ (grey bars) and SPC-GM (black bars) mice were determined by flow cytometry. (A) AEC II proportion of lung homogenate cells; bar graphs represent the percentage of pro-SP-C$^+$ cells in lung homogenates from n=3 mice per group. (B) Flow-cytometric analysis of AEC I (T1-α$^+$) percentage in lung homogenates of untreated and LPS-treated mice. (C) Total AEC (AEC II + AEC I) numbers in lung homogenates before and after 96 h of LPS. Total AEC numbers were calculated from the respective AEC II and AEC I percentages and total cell numbers of homogenates. Data is given as means ± SD from n=3 mice per group. Values are given as means ± SD. **p<0.01, ***p<0.001.

Results

Given that epithelial GM-CSF contributed to AEC II proliferation in the resolution phase of LPS-induced lung injury, the contribution of epithelial GM-CSF in the restoration of alveolar barrier function in the LPS-model was subsequently investigated. Therefore, alveolar leakage was assessed in LPS-injured mice of the three treatment groups in the time course after LPS administration. A prominent induction of alveolar leakage in wt and SPC-GM mice after 6 h of LPS instillation was detected, which was found to be reduced to baseline levels after 96 h. $GM^{-/-}$ mice, however, showed a sustained increase of alveolar barrier dysfunction until 240 h post LPS administration, suggesting that GM-CSF, by enhancing AEC II proliferation and renewal, contributes to restoration of alveolar barrier function severely disturbed in LPS-induced acute lung injury (Fig. 27).

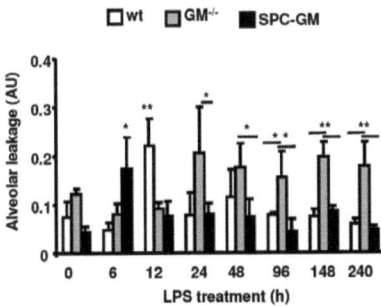

Figure 27. Alveolar leakage in wt (white bars), $GM^{-/-}$ (grey bars) and SPC-GM (black bars) at various time intervals post LPS administration. Data is given as the ratio between FITC fluorescence in BALF and serum (arbitrary units, AU). Data is presented as means ± SD from at least n=3 animals per group; *p<0.05, **p<0.01.

To investigate whether the observed influence of pro-inflammatory activated AMφ in alveolar epithelial repair in the LPS model also occurred in Gram-negative pneumonia, wt mice were intratracheally treated with *K. pneumoniae* for the indicated time intervals and total BALF leukocyte numbers were analysed and differential counts performed. As demonstrated in Fig. 28, *K. pneumoniae* infection in wt mice resulted in a similar, yet more severe inflammatory reaction compared to the LPS model, characterised by a high leukocyte influx 48 hours after infection (hpi), correlating with the neutrophil peak following infection. Similar to the findings in LPS-challenged mice, *K. pneumoniae* infection in wt mice resulted in a prominent production of GM-CSF and TNF-α at the early onset of inflammation (Fig. 29).

Results

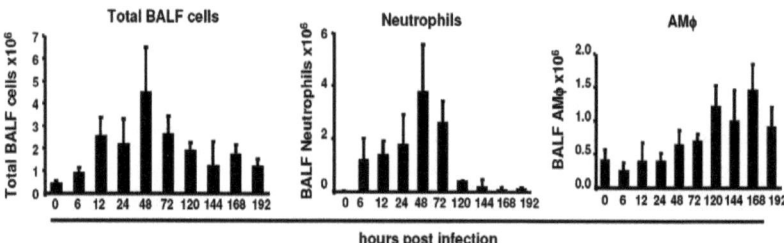

Figure 28. Quantification of total BALF leukocytes and leukocyte-subpopulations after *K. pneumoniae* infection in wt mice. BALF was performed at different time intervals post intratracheal infection with 25×10^4 CFU/mouse. Total BALF cell counts were determined and leukocyte differential counts were obtained from Pappenheim-stained cytocentrifuge preparations. Data is given as total cells and represents means ± SD from n=3 animals per group.

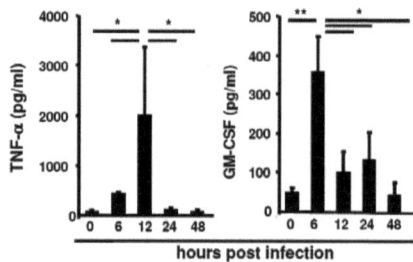

Figure 29. TNF-α and GM-CSF levels in BALF from *K. pneumoniae* infected wt mice. Data is presented as means ± SD from n=3 mice per group; *p<0.05, **p<0.01.

Resembling the LPS-model, the cytokine release correlated with an increased proliferation of AEC II at 72 h post *K. pneumoniae* infection, which thereafter gradually decreased until 192 hpi (Fig. 30A). Furthermore, the AEC II proportion in lung homogenates decreased at 72 hpi most likely due to AEC II injury, but was steadily replenished until 192 hpi (Fig. 30B). In addition, intraalveolar TNF-α neutralisation 72 hpi resulted in a remarkable decrease of AEC II proliferation, as well as decrease of the AEC II proportion in lung homogenates (Fig. 30C).

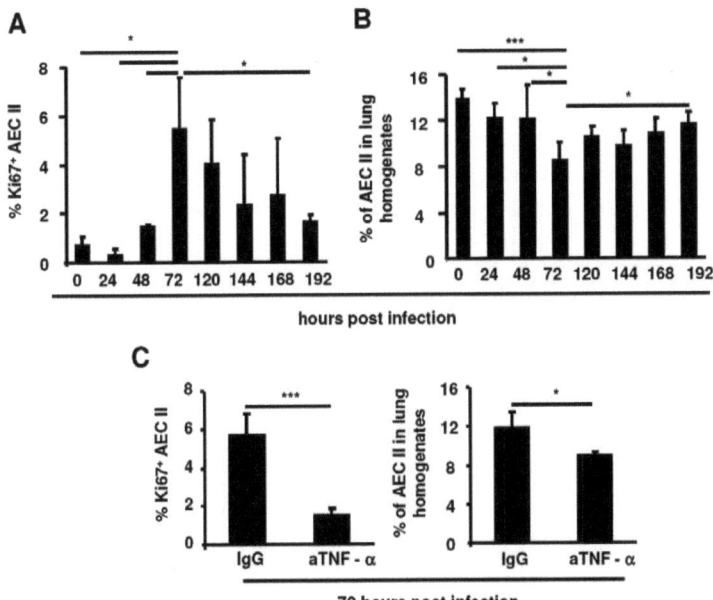

Figure 30. Alveolar repair after *K. pneumoniae* infection is associated with TNF-α-dependent AEC II proliferation. (A) At the indicated time points the proliferating proportion of AEC II was determined in *K. pneumoniae* infected mice. Bar graphs represent the percentage of Ki67$^+$ of total AEC II (pro SP-C$^+$/CD45$^-$) in lung homogenates from n=3 mice per group. (B) AEC II proportion (pro SP-C$^+$) of lung homogenate cells from lavaged lungs of n=3 mice per group. (C) FACS quantification of proliferating AEC II *(left panel)* and AEC II proportion in lung homogenates *(right panel)* of wt mice (n=3) infected intratracheally with *K. pneumoniae* and treated with either a-TNF-α or respective IgG antibodies, for 72 h. Values are means ± SD. *p<0.05, ***p<0.001.

5. Discussion

Damage of the endo-epithelial barrier is the major hallmark of acute lung injury upon bacterial infection, associated with oedema formation, alveolar flooding, impaired fluid clearance and gas exchange. Hence, to restore the normal lung function, alveolar repair processes are ultimately initiated (34). Resident alveolar macrophages have been assigned a contributing role in epithelial repair, closely associated with the transition of the pro-inflammatory into the anti-inflammatory macrophage phenotype (62, 94). In the current thesis the potential of early activated, pro-inflammatory resident alveolar macrophages to influence epithelial repair processes was investigated. Moreover, the hypothesis that pro-inflammatory resident alveolar macrophages may contribute to effective epithelial repair after LPS- and *K. pneumoniae* induced lung injury was tested. Hence, *in vitro* experiments revealed that alveolar epithelial cells co-cultured with LPS-stimulated resident alveolar macrophages express significantly higher amounts of growth factors, particularly of GM-CSF. Macrophage TNF-α released upon LPS stimulation was identified as a mediator inducing GM-CSF expression in epithelial cells, which in turn elicited autocrine proliferative signalling in type II alveolar epithelial cells. Genetic deletion of GM-CSF resulted in absence of macrophage-induced epithelial cell proliferation. Similarly, *in vivo* TNF-α neutralization after LPS-induced lung injury impaired epithelial proliferation. Furthermore, GM-CSF-deficient mice displayed reduced AEC II proliferation and sustained alveolar leakage after LPS challenge. Similarly, *K. pneumoniae*-induced lung injury was associated with early release of TNF-α and GM-CSF, and subsequent TNF-α-dependent AEC II proliferation during the alveolar repair phase. Altogether, these data reveal that alveolar repair processes are initiated early in the inflammatory course of pathogen-induced acute lung injury, and are mediated by macrophage TNF-α and epithelial GM-CSF (Fig. 31).

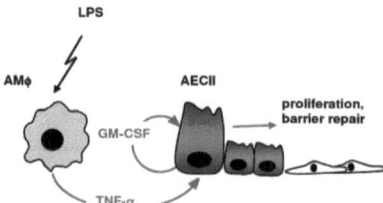

Figure 31. Proposed model of AMϕ/AEC cross-talk in alveolar barrier repair. TNF-α released from LPS-activated AMϕ induces expression of GM-CSF in alveolar epithelial cells, which in turn mediates AEC II proliferation and barrier renewal via a STAT5-dependent autocrine signalling loop.

Discussion

5.1. The contribution of pro-inflammatory resident alveolar macrophages to epithelial repair

Alveolar macrophages at the site of inflammation have been demonstrated to acquire an anti-inflammatory phenotype driven by lipid mediator-induced signalling, and hence to actively promote the resolution of inflammation. These signalling events trigger increased macrophage phagocytosis activity, decreased neutrophil migration, diminished superoxide production by neutrophils and iNOS by macrophages, as well as reduced adhesion molecule activation and gene expression (102). Additionally, the decreased NF-κB activation in alveolar macrophages results in a profile switch of released cytokines, from pro- to anti-inflammatory mediators such as TGF-ß and IL-10 (62). Moreover, previous reports demonstrated that anti-inflammatory AMϕ directly release epithelial mitogens, thereby inducing alveolar epithelial cell proliferation (60, 61, 103). The current data add to the aforementioned concept of macrophage-epithelial cross-talk during alveolar reparative events. Interestingly, the present thesis evidences that LPS-activated AMϕ, via release of the pro-inflammatory cytokine TNF-α, have the potential to stimulate AEC themselves to produce epithelial growth factors, thereby enhancing alveolar repair processes. In contrast, LPS-activated AMϕ did not express any of the epithelial mitogens analysed, implying that pro-inflammatory AMϕ most likely indirectly initiate epithelial repair signalling via soluble mediators. Hence, this thesis provided data demonstrating that alveolar epithelial cell proliferation is dependent on macrophage TNF-α *in vitro* and *in vivo*. Of note, our group recently showed that "exudate macrophages" (ExMϕ) massively recruited during influenza virus pneumonia may induce alveolar epithelial apoptosis via TNF-related apoptosis inducing ligand (TRAIL), thereby contributing to loss of barrier function (87). In contrast, in the LPS-model with very limited ExMϕ accumulation in the airspaces ($0.0565 \pm 0.02 \times 10^6$ after 96 h), opposing reparative effects of AMϕ towards the alveolar epithelium were observed. Such a divergent role of lung macrophages emerges most likely from the macrophage phenotype analysed (resident vs. recruited) and the different inflammatory models applied.

TNF-α is an early pro-inflammatory cytokine, known to be primarily released from activated resident alveolar macrophages and to stimulate alveolar cell populations for chemokine release and adhesion molecule expression, thereby initiating and maintaining innate host defence (43). Besides its predominant pro-inflammatory, tissue-destructive role, several reports suggested TNF-α to exert resolution- and repair-enhancing effects by different mechanisms. In this line, TNF-α was shown to induce urokinase-type plasminogen activator in alveolar epithelial cells followed by lysis of alveolar fibrin and resolution of inflammation (104). Similar to the data presented in the current thesis, TNF-α was described as a mediator of the proliferation of gastric epithelium and human retinal pigment epithelial cells (65, 105). Moreover, TNF-α has been previously reported to induce expression of GM-CSF in endothelial cells and fibroblasts via activation and nuclear translocation of the transcription factor NF-κB (67, 106). Furthermore, NF-κB was shown to be nuclearly translocated upon TNF receptor binding in human lung epithelial cells (107). Besides its widely known pro-inflammatory function, NFκB has recently been associated with signalling events mediating the resolution of inflammation, particularly via TGF-ß1 production (108), thereby strengthening the concept of a dichotomic role of TNF-α induced signalling events in acute inflammation.

Taken together, the data presented in this thesis suggest that epithelial repair processes are implemented yet in the acute phase of alveolar inflammation and highlight the complexity of intercellular communication in lung inflammation and repair.

5.2. GM-CSF induced proliferative signalling in AEC

The current thesis evidenced that TNF-α-mediated alveolar epithelial cell proliferation was largely mediated by the epithelial growth factor GM-CSF *in vitro* and *in vivo*. GM-CSF is a well known growth factor for phagocytes, but it also stimulates maturation of eosinophils, erythrocytes, megakaryocytes and dendritic cells. Apart from its effects on progenitor cells, GM-CSF improves host defence functions of mature hematopoietic cells, such as alveolar macrophages (68). More recent reports suggested a role of GM-CSF in the proliferation of alveolar type II cells (75, 77), however, the contribution of GM-CSF to epithelial repair and restoration of alveolar barrier function upon LPS-induced acute lung injury has not previously been addressed.

Murine alveolar epithelial cells type II were shown to express the GM-CSF receptor α–subunit on lung tissue sections, whereas both α and ß subunits have been identified on freshly isolated rat AEC II (75, 76). Likewise, the data presented in this thesis demonstrated that both subunits are expressed in freshly isolated murine alveolar epithelial cells and downregulated during 5 days of *in vitro* trans-differentiation into type I-like cells, which was associated with pronounced proliferation of AEC at day 1, but not at day 3 of culture upon GM-CSF stimulation. Our group and others have observed that freshly isolated AEC in culture rapidly lose the type II phenotype (in less then 24 h), which is the major limit of the *in*

Discussion

vitro studies with these cells (25, 109). In order to overcome this problem, a previously described *in vitro* model to preserve the AEC type II phenotype during culture was used (25). Accordingly, freshly isolated murine AEC were grown for up to 3 days on matrigel:collagen matrix. Under these conditions, differentiation was significantly diminished and the majority of the cells retained the "classical" type II phenotype. AEC cultured on matrigel:collagen matrix proliferated in response to GM-CSF and co-culture with LPS-stimulated AMϕ revealed epithelial release of GM-CSF associated with increased AEC proliferation, thus confirming the concept that type II cells as opposed to type I cells represent the proliferating subpopulation (6).
Furthermore additional evidence is provided that GM-CSF-induced alveolar epithelial cell proliferation was signalled by STAT5 phosphorylation resulting in increased expression of Cyclin D1. The JAK2-STAT5-Cyclin D1 pathway has been shown to be the underlying mechanism in prolactin stimulated proliferation of mammary epithelial cells (101). Of note, GM-CSF-mediated activation of cellular repair mechanisms has been similarly evidenced in different cell types such as endothelial cells and keratinocytes, resulting in increased proliferation and subsequently enhanced *in vivo* angiogenesis and wound healing (110, 111). Despite the fact that the JAK2-STAT5 axis has been evidenced to influence the cellular differentiation and phenotype (112), a non significant influence of GM-CSF signalling on the process of AEC II to I differentiation *in vitro* was identified. Interestingly, GM-CSF activation of JAK2 and STAT5 in human monocytes has been associated with induction of CCL2 production (99). In contrast, GM-CSF-stimulated AEC in the presented study did not reveal increased pro-inflammatory chemokine production. Additionally, GM-CSF was reported to activate MAPK and PI3K in myeloid cells (100), however activation of these pathways in alveolar epithelial cells was not detected.
In summary, GM-CSF stimulation induced proliferative signalling in alveolar epithelial cells, most likely dependent on intracellular STAT5 activation and Cyclin D1 induction.

5.3. The role of the TNF-α – GM-CSF axis in alveolar repair following acute lung injury

Given that the *in vitro* study revealed macrophage-TNF-α induced expression of GM-CSF in AEC, followed by an autocrine proliferative signalling, it was subsequently investigated whether a similar mechanism may drive the alveolar epithelial repair *in vivo*, in an LPS and *K. pneumoniae* model of acute lung injury.

Discussion

In accordance with data obtained from a rat model (8), the current thesis demonstrated that alveolar repair processes in terms of epithelial cell type II proliferation were initiated 4 days after LPS instillation, when alveolar inflammation decreased virtually to baseline levels. In contrast, a significantly reduced epithelial proliferation and sustained loss of barrier function throughout day 10 post LPS challenge was observed in GM-CSF-deficient mice *in vivo*, confirming the *in vitro* findings with GM-CSF-deficient alveolar epithelial cells lacking a TNF-α-induced proliferative response. Interestingly, AEC II proliferation after LPS challenge was completely rescued in SPC-GM mice, and epithelial GM-CSF release was widely reduced upon alveolar TNF-α neutralisation in wt mice *in vivo*. These data clearly indicate that the alveolar epithelium itself is the primary source of GM-CSF, which is in turn released in the presence of TNF-α, emphasizing the central role of alveolar type II epithelial cells in perpetuating self-renewal and barrier restoration once they have received an initial macrophage signal.

Interestingly, the neutrophilic response in $GM^{-/-}$ mice was more pronounced at 6 to 24 hours after LPS treatment as compared to wt mice, correlating with the previous findings that $GM^{-/-}$ neutrophils are fully functional and their recruitment at the onset of inflammation is successfully (over-)compensated (113). Moreover, Paine *et al* evidenced a decreased activity of $GM^{-/-}$ alveolar macrophages characterised with impaired *in vitro* phagocytosis and decreased TNF-α release, which *in vivo* resulted in increased susceptibility to *Pneumocystis carinii* infection and increased inflammation, compared to wild-type mice (114). Therefore, it was assumed that the prolonged alveolar neutrophil presence observed at 96 and 148 h post LPS instillation is most likely due to alveolar macrophage dysfunction in $GM^{-/-}$ mice with decreased phagocytosis of apoptotic neutrophils and delayed resolution of alveolar inflammation.

Alveolar barrier disruption has been described as a neutrophil-mediated damage resulting in paracellular permeability, which in turn leads to leakage of fluids that characterize the acute lung injury (ALI). At least three distinct mechanisms are involved in opening the epithelium: (1) highly regulated disassembly and reassembly of tight junctions, (2) mechanical force resulting in epithelial wounds, especially during high tidal volume ventilation, and (3) degradative effects of neutrophil derived mediators (pro-apoptotic factors, proteases or reactive oxygen/nitrogen species) (115, 116). Importantly, in the presented thesis, sustained lung leakage in $GM^{-/-}$ mice was observed beyond the neutrophil decrease (240 h) indicating that the inflammatory injured epithelial barrier lacked an adequate proliferation stimulus in absence of GM-CSF. In contrast, neutrophil clearance was enhanced in GM-CSF-

Discussion

overexpressing (SPC-GM) mice, most likely correlated to increased GM-CSF amounts in BALF and subsequently enhanced macrophage phagocytotic function. SPC-GM mice also displayed faster alveolar neutrophilic influx than wt mice, probably due to the chemotactic activity of GM-CSF taking effects when present in excessive amounts (117).

Alveolar TNF-α levels peaked at 6 h post LPS instillation in all treatment groups, however they were significantly increased in SPC-GM mice and decreased in GM-CSF-deficient compared to wt mice, indicating that, apart from its reparative effects on epithelial cells, GM-CSF may enhance macrophage host defence functions. A recent report suggested that GM-CSF regulates TLR4-dependent signalling events such as TNF-α release from LPS-treated alveolar macrophages via activation of the transcription factor PU.1 (118). Therefore, GM-CSF might promote alveolar repair upon bacterial pneumonia in two ways: first, due to its direct proliferative effects on alveolar epithelium, and second, by enhancing macrophage TNF-α release, which in turn mediates further epithelial GM-CSF expression. TNF-α inhibition as therapeutic strategy to attenuate acute or chronic pulmonary inflammation might therefore hold the risk of insufficient tissue repair.

Although recognition of LPS by TLR4 is an essential step in initiating an effective immune response in gram-negative pneumonia (119, 120), LPS instillation alone does not fully reflect the complex events observed in bacterial pneumonia. Hence, a *K. pneumoniae* pneumonia model was used to evaluate the role of macrophage – epithelial cross-talk during the alveolar repair phase after acute gram-negative pneumonia. The presented data confirm that macrophage TNF-α is indeed a crucial mediator initiating AEC II proliferation during *K. pneumoniae* infection.

Taken together, the current thesis demonstrates that epithelial repair processes may be primed already in the pro-inflammatory phase of acute lung injury. Novel evidence is provided for the key role of macrophage TNF-α inducing alveolar repair via epithelial GM-CSF. Thus, detection of distinct intercellular cross-talk mechanisms mediating tissue repair in the course of severe pneumonia may identify therapeutic targets allowing timed and compartment-specific intervention strategies promoting regeneration of the injured alveolar barrier.

6. Summary

Bacterial invasion of the alveolar air space is followed by the fast, tightly regulated immune response facilitating a successful pathogen clearance. Upon pathogen recognition activated resident alveolar macrophages (AMφ) early release pro-inflammatory cytokines, stimulating neighbouring alveolar cells to produce chemokines which in turn mediate the infiltration of neutrophils, exudate macrophages and lymphocytes. The following inflammatory reaction and the pathogen itself leave a damaged alveolar barrier associated with pulmonary oedema and impaired gas exchange. Consequently, epithelial repair processes are initiated to restore the normal lung homeostasis. During the later phase of infection AMφ have been shown to acquire an anti-inflammatory phenotype thereby enhancing alveolar repair processes. However, the potential of early activated, pro-inflammatory AMφ to influence epithelial repair remains largely elusive. Therefore, in the present thesis it was investigated whether activated AMφ contribute to alveolar epithelial repair upon LPS challenge *in vitro* and *in vivo*, as well as in *K. pneumoniae* pneumonia, and the molecular interaction pathways involved were analysed. The cross-talk between resident alveolar macrophages and alveolar epithelial cells during alveolar repair was assessed in an *in vitro* co-culture system and an *in vivo* model of LPS-induced acute lung injury. Gene expression and protein analysis showed that LPS-activated alveolar macrophages stimulated alveolar epithelial cells (AEC) to express growth factors, particularly GM-CSF upon co-culture. Antibody neutralization experiments revealed epithelial GM-CSF expression to be macrophage TNF-α dependent. GM-CSF elicited proliferative signalling in alveolar epithelial cells via autocrine activation of the transcription factor STAT 5 and Cyclin D1 expression. Notably, macrophage TNF-α induced epithelial proliferation in wild-type but not in GM-CSF-deficient alveolar epithelial cells as shown by [^{3}H]-thymidine incorporation and cell counting. Matrigel:collagen AEC culture preserving the type II phenotype *in vitro* supported the concept that the proliferative response to GM-CSF is related to the type II AEC phenotype. Moreover, intra-alveolar TNF-α neutralization impaired alveolar epithelial type II cell proliferation in LPS-injured mice *in vivo*, as investigated by flow cytometric Ki67 and immunofluorescence staining of lung sections. Additionally, GM-CSF-deficient mice displayed reduced AEC II proliferation and sustained alveolar barrier dysfunction upon LPS treatment compared to wild-type and SPC-GM mice (overexpressing GM-CSF in AEC II in a GM-CSF-deficient background). Similarly, *K. pneumoniae* lung infection confirmed the findings in the LPS-model and resulted in early release of macrophage

Summary

TNF-α and epithelial GM-CSF, as well as subsequent TNF-α-dependent AEC II proliferation during alveolar repair events.

Collectively, these findings indicate that TNF-α released from activated resident alveolar macrophages induces epithelial GM-CSF expression, which in turn initiates alveolar epithelial type II cell proliferation and thus contributes to restore alveolar barrier function.

7. Zusammenfassung

Die bakterielle Infektion des Alveolarraumes ist regelhaft von einer schnellen, streng koordinierten Immunantwort gefolgt, deren Ziel die rasche Elimination des Erregers ist. Nach der Erkennung des Erregers über spezielle Pathogen-Rezeptoren setzen Alveolarmakrophagen (AMΦ) pro-inflammatorische Zytokine frei und stimulieren benachbarte Parenchymzellen zur Produktion von Chemokinen, welche letztendlich die Chemotaxis neutrophiler Granulozyten, von Exudatmakrophagen und Lymphozyten vermitteln. Diese Immunreaktion, aber auch die Infektion selbst, führen zu einer Destruktion der alveolären Barriere mit konsekutivem alveolärem Ödem und eingeschränktem Gasaustausch. In der Folge werden alveoläre Reparaturprozesse in Gang gesetzt, um die Organfunktion wieder herzustellen. Alveolarmakrophagen aquirieren in der Spätphase der Entzündung einen anti-inflammatorischen Phänotyp und können solche Reparaturprozesse in Gang setzen. Jedoch war das Reparaturpotenzial früh aktivierter, pro-inflammatorischer Alveolarmakrophagen bis dato ungeklärt. In der vorliegenden Arbeit wurde deshalb untersucht, ob früh-inflammatorisch aktivierte residente Alveolarmakrophagen zur alveolarepithelialen Reparatur nach LPS-Applikation *in vitro* und *in vivo* und im *Klebsiella*-Pneumonie-Modell beitragen und welche die zugrunde liegenden molekularen Mechanismen sind. Es wurden die Mediatoren des Cross-talk zwischen Alveolarmakrophagen und Alveolarepithel in der alveolarepithelialen Reparatur in einem *in vitro* Ko-Kulturmodell und im Mausmodell der LPS-induzierten Acute Lung Injury ermittelt. Genexpressions- und Proteinanalysen zeigten hierbei, dass LPS-aktivierte Alveolarmakrophagen in der Ko-Kultur Alveolarepithelzellen zur Freisetzung epithelialer Wachstumsfaktoren, insbesondere von GM-CSF, stimulieren. Neutralisationsexperimente zeigten, dass die epitheliale GM-CSF Expression abhängig war von Makrophagen-sezerniertem TNF-α. GM-CSF induzierte autokrin eine STAT5-Cyclin D1-vermittelte proliferative Signalkaskade in Alveolarepithelzellen. Interessanterweise konnte mittels [^{3}H]-Thymidin-Einbau und Zellzählung gezeigt werden, dass TNF-α eine epitheliale Proliferation in Wildtyp-, nicht jedoch in GM-CSF-defizienten Alveolarepithelzellen induziert. Ähnliche Experimente mit Alveolarepithelzellen, die auf einer Matrigel:Collagen-Matrix kultiviert wurden und dabei einen Phänotyp II (AEC II) behielten, zeigten, dass diese GM-CSF-vermittelte Proliferationsantwort an den Phänotyp II gekoppelt war. Darüberhinaus konnte im LPS-Mausmodell gezeigt werden, dass die intraalveoläre Neutralisation von TNF-α die Proliferation von Typ II Alveolarepithelzellen *in vivo*, gemessen anhand der Ki-67 Expression im FACS und in der Immunfluoreszenz, deutlich reduzierte. Zusätzlich zeigten GM-CSF-defiziente Mäuse eine eingeschränkte Alveolarepithelzellproliferation und eine

Summary

deutlich prolongierte Dysfunktion der alveolären Barriere nach intratrachealer LPS-Gabe verglichen mit Wildtyp- oder SPC-GM-Mäusen (mit Überexpression von GM-CSF im Alveolarepithel, generiert in GM-CSF-defizienten Mäusen). Im *Klebsiella*-Pneumoniemodell konnten diese Mechanismen bestätigt werden. Zusammenfassend konnte gezeigt werden, dass TNF-α, welches von LPS-aktivierten residenten Alveolarmakrophagen freigesetzt wird, eine alveolarepitheliale GM-CSF-Expression induziert. GM-CSF wiederum initiiert über eine autokrine Signalkaskade die Proliferation von Typ II Alveolarepithelzellen und trägt somit wesentlich zur Erneuerung und Funktionalität der alveolarepithelialen Barriere bei.

8. References

1. Cell-Culture Models of Biological Barriers. In vitro Test-systems for Drug Absorption and Delivery. Routledge, USA.
2. Bastacky, J., Lee C. Y., Goerke J., Koushafar H., Yager D., Kenaga L., Speed T. P., Chen Y., and Clements J. A. 1995. Alveolar lining layer is thin and continuous: low-temperature scanning electron microscopy of rat lung. *J Appl Physiol* 79(5):1615-28.
3. von Wulffen, W., Steinmueller M., Herold S., Marsh L. M., Bulau P., Seeger W., Welte T., Lohmeyer J., and Maus U. A. 2007. Lung dendritic cells elicited by Fms-like tyrosine 3-kinase ligand amplify the lung inflammatory response to lipopolysaccharide. *Am J Respir Crit Care Med* 176(9):892-901.
4. Mason, R. J., Williams M. C., Greenleaf R. D., and Clements J. A. 1977. Isolation and properties of type II alveolar cells from rat lung. *Am Rev Respir Dis* 115(6):1015-26.
5. Beers, M. F., Kim C. Y., Dodia C., and Fisher A. B. 1994. Localization, synthesis, and processing of surfactant protein SP-C in rat lung analyzed by epitope-specific antipeptide antibodies. *J Biol Chem* 269(32):20318-28.
6. Fehrenbach, H. 2001. Alveolar epithelial type II cell: defender of the alveolus revisited. *Respir Res* 2(1):33-46.
7. Phelps, D. S., and Floros J. 1991. Localization of pulmonary surfactant proteins using immunohistochemistry and tissue in situ hybridization. *Exp Lung Res* 17(6):985-95.
8. Berthiaume, Y., Lesur O., and Dagenais A. 1999. Treatment of adult respiratory distress syndrome: plea for rescue therapy of the alveolar epithelium. *Thorax* 54(2):150-60.
9. Matthay, M. A., Robriquet L., and Fang X. 2005. Alveolar epithelium: role in lung fluid balance and acute lung injury. *Proc Am Thorac Soc* 2(3):206-13.
10. Stephens, R. H., Benjamin A. R., and Walters D. V. 1996. Volume and protein concentration of epithelial lining liquid in perfused in situ postnatal sheep lungs. *J Appl Physiol* 80(6):1911-20.
11. Adamson, I. Y., and Bowden D. H. 1974. The type 2 cell as progenitor of alveolar epithelial regeneration. A cytodynamic study in mice after exposure to oxygen. *Lab Invest* 30(1):35-42.
12. Clegg, G. R., Tyrrell C., McKechnie S. R., Beers M. F., Harrison D., and McElroy M. C. 2005. Coexpression of RTI40 with alveolar epithelial type II cell proteins in lungs following injury: identification of alveolar intermediate cell types. *Am J Physiol Lung Cell Mol Physiol* 289(3):L382-90.
13. Evans, M. J., Cabral L. J., Stephens R. J., and Freeman G. 1973. Renewal of alveolar epithelium in the rat following exposure to NO2. *Am J Pathol* 70(2):175-98.
14. Williams, M. C. 2003. Alveolar type I cells: molecular phenotype and development. *Annu Rev Physiol* 65:669-95.
15. Uhal, B. D. 1997. Cell cycle kinetics in the alveolar epithelium. *Am J Physiol* 272(6 Pt 1):L1031-45.
16. Kalina, M., Riklis S., and Blau H. 1993. Pulmonary epithelial cell proliferation in primary culture of alveolar type II cells. *Exp Lung Res* 19(2):153-75.

References

17. Reddy, R., Buckley S., Doerken M., Barsky L., Weinberg K., Anderson K. D., Warburton D., and Driscoll B. 2004. Isolation of a putative progenitor subpopulation of alveolar epithelial type 2 cells. *Am J Physiol Lung Cell Mol Physiol* 286(4):L658-67.
18. Berthiaume, Y., Voisin G., and Dagenais A. 2006. The alveolar type I cells: the new knight of the alveolus? *J Physiol* 572(Pt 3):609-10.
19. Weibel, E. R. 1971. The mystery of "non-nucleated plates" in the alveolar epithelium of the lung explained. *Acta Anat (Basel)* 78(3):425-43.
20. McElroy, M. C., and Kasper M. 2004. The use of alveolar epithelial type I cell-selective markers to investigate lung injury and repair. *Eur Respir J* 24(4):664-73.
21. Borok, Z., Li X., Fernandes V. F., Zhou B., Ann D. K., and Crandall E. D. 2000. Differential regulation of rat aquaporin-5 promoter/enhancer activities in lung and salivary epithelial cells. *J Biol Chem* 275(34):26507-14.
22. Johnson, M. D., Bao H. F., Helms M. N., Chen X. J., Tigue Z., Jain L., Dobbs L. G., and Eaton D. C. 2006. Functional ion channels in pulmonary alveolar type I cells support a role for type I cells in lung ion transport. *Proc Natl Acad Sci U S A* 103(13):4964-9.
23. Shannon, J. M., Jennings S. D., and Nielsen L. D. 1992. Modulation of alveolar type II cell differentiated function in vitro. *Am J Physiol* 262(4 Pt 1):L427-36.
24. Borok, Z., Danto S. I., Lubman R. L., Cao Y., Williams M. C., and Crandall E. D. 1998. Modulation of t1alpha expression with alveolar epithelial cell phenotype in vitro. *Am J Physiol* 275(1 Pt 1):L155-64.
25. Rice, W. R., Conkright J. J., Na C. L., Ikegami M., Shannon J. M., and Weaver T. E. 2002. Maintenance of the mouse type II cell phenotype in vitro. *Am J Physiol Lung Cell Mol Physiol* 283(2):L256-64.
26. Wang, J., Edeen K., Manzer R., Chang Y., Wang S., Chen X., Funk C. J., Cosgrove G. P., Fang X., and Mason R. J. 2007. Differentiated human alveolar epithelial cells and reversibility of their phenotype in vitro. *Am J Respir Cell Mol Biol* 36(6):661-8.
27. Bhaskaran, M., Kolliputi N., Wang Y., Gou D., Chintagari N. R., and Liu L. 2007. Trans-differentiation of alveolar epithelial type II cells to type I cells involves autocrine signaling by transforming growth factor beta 1 through the Smad pathway. *J Biol Chem* 282(6):3968-76.
28. Qiao, R., Yan W., Clavijo C., Mehrian-Shai R., Zhong Q., Kim K. J., Ann D., Crandall E. D., and Borok Z. 2008. Effects of KGF on alveolar epithelial cell transdifferentiation are mediated by JNK signaling. *Am J Respir Cell Mol Biol* 38(2):239-46.
29. Chen, J., Chen Z., Narasaraju T., Jin N., and Liu L. 2004. Isolation of highly pure alveolar epithelial type I and type II cells from rat lungs. *Lab Invest* 84(6):727-35.
30. Martin, T. R., and Frevert C. W. 2005. Innate immunity in the lungs. *Proc Am Thorac Soc* 2(5):403-11.
31. Delclaux, C., and Azoulay E. 2003. Inflammatory response to infectious pulmonary injury. *Eur Respir J Suppl* 42:10s-14s.
32. Lee, W. L., and Downey G. P. 2001. Neutrophil activation and acute lung injury. *Curr Opin Crit Care* 7(1):1-7.
33. Wang, H. M., Bodenstein M., and Markstaller K. 2008. Overview of the pathology of three widely used animal models of acute lung injury. *Eur Surg Res* 40(4):305-16.

References

34. Ware, L. B., and Matthay M. A. 2000. The acute respiratory distress syndrome. *N Engl J Med* 342(18):1334-49.

35. Kelley, J. 1990. Cytokines of the lung. *Am Rev Respir Dis* 141(3):765-88.

36. Toews, G. B. 2001. Cytokines and the lung. *Eur Respir J Suppl* 34:3s-17s.

37. Vanderbilt, J. N., Mager E. M., Allen L., Sawa T., Wiener-Kronish J., Gonzalez R., and Dobbs L. G. 2003. CXC chemokines and their receptors are expressed in type II cells and upregulated following lung injury. *Am J Respir Cell Mol Biol* 29(6):661-8.

38. Delves, P. J., and Roitt I. M. 2000. The immune system. First of two parts. *N Engl J Med* 343(1):37-49.

39. Maus, U. A., Janzen S., Wall G., Srivastava M., Blackwell T. S., Christman J. W., Seeger W., Welte T., and Lohmeyer J. 2006. Resident alveolar macrophages are replaced by recruited monocytes in response to endotoxin-induced lung inflammation. *Am J Respir Cell Mol Biol* 35(2):227-35.

40. Diamond, G., Legarda D., and Ryan L. K. 2000. The innate immune response of the respiratory epithelium. *Immunol Rev* 173:27-38.

41. MacRedmond, R., Greene C., Taggart C. C., McElvaney N., and O'Neill S. 2005. Respiratory epithelial cells require Toll-like receptor 4 for induction of human beta-defensin 2 by lipopolysaccharide. *Respir Res* 6:116.

42. Golec, M. 2007. Cathelicidin LL-37: LPS-neutralizing, pleiotropic peptide. *Ann Agric Environ Med* 14(1):1-4.

43. Herold, S., von Wulffen W., Steinmueller M., Pleschka S., Kuziel W. A., Mack M., Srivastava M., Seeger W., Maus U. A., and Lohmeyer J. 2006. Alveolar epithelial cells direct monocyte transepithelial migration upon influenza virus infection: impact of chemokines and adhesion molecules. *J Immunol* 177(3):1817-24.

44. Serhan, C. N., Chiang N., and Van Dyke T. E. 2008. Resolving inflammation: dual anti-inflammatory and pro-resolution lipid mediators. *Nat Rev Immunol* 8(5):349-61.

45. Serhan, C. N., Brain S. D., Buckley C. D., Gilroy D. W., Haslett C., O'Neill L. A., Perretti M., Rossi A. G., and Wallace J. L. 2007. Resolution of inflammation: state of the art, definitions and terms. *Faseb J* 21(2):325-32.

46. Serhan, C. N. 2004. A search for endogenous mechanisms of anti-inflammation uncovers novel chemical mediators: missing links to resolution. *Histochem Cell Biol* 122(4):305-21.

47. Levy, B. D., Clish C. B., Schmidt B., Gronert K., and Serhan C. N. 2001. Lipid mediator class switching during acute inflammation: signals in resolution. *Nat Immunol* 2(7):612-9.

48. Freire-de-Lima, C. G., Xiao Y. Q., Gardai S. J., Bratton D. L., Schiemann W. P., and Henson P. M. 2006. Apoptotic cells, through transforming growth factor-beta, coordinately induce anti-inflammatory and suppress pro-inflammatory eicosanoid and NO synthesis in murine macrophages. *J Biol Chem* 281(50):38376-84.

49. Serhan, C. N., Hong S., Gronert K., Colgan S. P., Devchand P. R., Mirick G., and Moussignac R. L. 2002. Resolvins: a family of bioactive products of omega-3 fatty acid transformation circuits initiated by aspirin treatment that counter proinflammation signals. *J Exp Med* 196(8):1025-37.

References

50. Campbell, E. L., Louis N. A., Tomassetti S. E., Canny G. O., Arita M., Serhan C. N., and Colgan S. P. 2007. Resolvin E1 promotes mucosal surface clearance of neutrophils: a new paradigm for inflammatory resolution. *Faseb J* 21(12):3162-70.
51. Filer, A., Pitzalis C., and Buckley C. D. 2006. Targeting the stromal microenvironment in chronic inflammation. *Curr Opin Pharmacol* 6(4):393-400.
52. Lesur, O., Arsalane K., and Lane D. 1996. Lung alveolar epithelial cell migration in vitro: modulators and regulation processes. *Am J Physiol* 270(3 Pt 1):L311-9.
53. Chesnutt, A. N., Kheradmand F., Folkesson H. G., Alberts M., and Matthay M. A. 1997. Soluble transforming growth factor-alpha is present in the pulmonary edema fluid of patients with acute lung injury. *Chest* 111(3):652-6.
54. Yanagita, K., Matsumoto K., Sekiguchi K., Ishibashi H., Niho Y., and Nakamura T. 1993. Hepatocyte growth factor may act as a pulmotrophic factor on lung regeneration after acute lung injury. *J Biol Chem* 268(28):21212-7.
55. Lesur, O., Melloni B., Cantin A. M., and Begin R. 1992. Silica-exposed lung fluids have a proliferative activity for type II epithelial cells: a study on human and sheep alveolar fluids. *Exp Lung Res* 18(5):633-54.
56. Fadok, V. A., Bratton D. L., Konowal A., Freed P. W., Westcott J. Y., and Henson P. M. 1998. Macrophages that have ingested apoptotic cells in vitro inhibit proinflammatory cytokine production through autocrine/paracrine mechanisms involving TGF-beta, PGE2, and PAF. *J Clin Invest* 101(4):890-8.
57. Jakowlew, S. B., Mariano J. M., You L., and Mathias A. 1997. Differential regulation of protease and extracellular matrix protein expression by transforming growth factor-beta 1 in non-small cell lung cancer cells and normal human bronchial epithelial cells. *Biochim Biophys Acta* 1353(2):157-70.
58. Zambruno, G., Marchisio P. C., Marconi A., Vaschieri C., Melchiori A., Giannetti A., and De Luca M. 1995. Transforming growth factor-beta 1 modulates beta 1 and beta 5 integrin receptors and induces the de novo expression of the alpha v beta 6 heterodimer in normal human keratinocytes: implications for wound healing. *J Cell Biol* 129(3):853-65.
59. Stiles, A. D., Smith B. T., and Post M. 1986. Reciprocal autocrine and paracrine regulation of growth of mesenchymal and alveolar epithelial cells from fetal lung. *Exp Lung Res* 11(3):165-77.
60. Melloni, B., Lesur O., Bouhadiba T., Cantin A., Martel M., and Begin R. 1996. Effect of exposure to silica on human alveolar macrophages in supporting growth activity in type II epithelial cells. *Thorax* 51(8):781-6.
61. Morimoto, K., Amano H., Sonoda F., Baba M., Senba M., Yoshimine H., Yamamoto H., Ii T., Oishi K., and Nagatake T. 2001. Alveolar macrophages that phagocytose apoptotic neutrophils produce hepatocyte growth factor during bacterial pneumonia in mice. *Am J Respir Cell Mol Biol* 24(5):608-15.
62. Duffield, J. S. 2003. The inflammatory macrophage: a story of Jekyll and Hyde. *Clin Sci (Lond)* 104(1):27-38.
63. Serhan, C. N., and Savill J. 2005. Resolution of inflammation: the beginning programs the end. *Nat Immunol* 6(12):1191-7.
64. Geiser, T., Jarreau P. H., Atabai K., and Matthay M. A. 2000. Interleukin-1beta augments in vitro alveolar epithelial repair. *Am J Physiol Lung Cell Mol Physiol* 279(6):L1184-90.

References

65. Luo, J. C., Shin V. Y., Yang Y. H., Wu W. K., Ye Y. N., So W. H., Chang F. Y., and Cho C. H. 2005. Tumor necrosis factor-alpha stimulates gastric epithelial cell proliferation. *Am J Physiol Gastrointest Liver Physiol* 288(1):G32-8.

66. Rezaiguia, S., Garat C., Delclaux C., Meignan M., Fleury J., Legrand P., Matthay M. A., and Jayr C. 1997. Acute bacterial pneumonia in rats increases alveolar epithelial fluid clearance by a tumor necrosis factor-alpha-dependent mechanism. *J Clin Invest* 99(2):325-35.

67. Gasson, J. C. 1991. Molecular physiology of granulocyte-macrophage colony-stimulating factor. *Blood* 77(6):1131-45.

68. Trapnell, B. C., and Whitsett J. A. 2002. Gm-CSF regulates pulmonary surfactant homeostasis and alveolar macrophage-mediated innate host defense. *Annu Rev Physiol* 64:775-802.

69. Gearing, D. P., Gough N. M., King J. A., Hilton D. J., Nicola N. A., Simpson R. J., Nice E. C., Kelso A., and Metcalf D. 1987. Molecular cloning and expression of cDNA encoding a murine myeloid leukaemia inhibitory factor (LIF). *Embo J* 6(13):3995-4002.

70. Hayashida, K., Kitamura T., Gorman D. M., Arai K., Yokota T., and Miyajima A. 1990. Molecular cloning of a second subunit of the receptor for human granulocyte-macrophage colony-stimulating factor (GM-CSF): reconstitution of a high-affinity GM-CSF receptor. *Proc Natl Acad Sci U S A* 87(24):9655-9.

71. Quelle, F. W., Sato N., Witthuhn B. A., Inhorn R. C., Eder M., Miyajima A., Griffin J. D., and Ihle J. N. 1994. JAK2 associates with the beta c chain of the receptor for granulocyte-macrophage colony-stimulating factor, and its activation requires the membrane-proximal region. *Mol Cell Biol* 14(7):4335-41.

72. Watanabe, S., Itoh T., and Arai K. 1996. Roles of JAK kinases in human GM-CSF receptor signal transduction. *J Allergy Clin Immunol* 98(6 Pt 2):S183-91.

73. Stanley, E., Lieschke G. J., Grail D., Metcalf D., Hodgson G., Gall J. A., Maher D. W., Cebon J., Sinickas V., and Dunn A. R. 1994. Granulocyte/macrophage colony-stimulating factor-deficient mice show no major perturbation of hematopoiesis but develop a characteristic pulmonary pathology. *Proc Natl Acad Sci U S A* 91(12):5592-6.

74. Dranoff, G., Crawford A. D., Sadelain M., Ream B., Rashid A., Bronson R. T., Dickersin G. R., Bachurski C. J., Mark E. L., Whitsett J. A., and et al. 1994. Involvement of granulocyte-macrophage colony-stimulating factor in pulmonary homeostasis. *Science* 264(5159):713-6.

75. Huffman Reed, J. A., Rice W. R., Zsengeller Z. K., Wert S. E., Dranoff G., and Whitsett J. A. 1997. GM-CSF enhances lung growth and causes alveolar type II epithelial cell hyperplasia in transgenic mice. *Am J Physiol* 273(4 Pt 1):L715-25.

76. Joshi, P. C., Applewhite L., Mitchell P. O., Fernainy K., Roman J., Eaton D. C., and Guidot D. M. 2006. GM-CSF receptor expression and signaling is decreased in lungs of ethanol-fed rats. *Am J Physiol Lung Cell Mol Physiol* 291(6):L1150-8.

77. Paine, R., 3rd, Wilcoxen S. E., Morris S. B., Sartori C., Baleeiro C. E., Matthay M. A., and Christensen P. J. 2003. Transgenic overexpression of granulocyte macrophage-colony stimulating factor in the lung prevents hyperoxic lung injury. *Am J Pathol* 163(6):2397-406.

78. Beck, J. M., Preston A. M., Wilcoxen S. E., Morris S. B., Sturrock A., and Paine R., 3rd. 2009. Critical roles of inflammation and apoptosis in improved survival in a model of hyperoxia-induced acute lung injury in Pneumocystis murina-infected mice. *Infect Immun* 77(3):1053-60.

References

79. Podschun, R., and Ullmann U. 1998. Klebsiella spp. as nosocomial pathogens: epidemiology, taxonomy, typing methods, and pathogenicity factors. *Clin Microbiol Rev* 11(4):589-603.

80. Royle, J., Halasz S., Eagles G., Gilbert G., Dalton D., Jelfs P., and Isaacs D. 1999. Outbreak of extended spectrum beta lactamase producing Klebsiella pneumoniae in a neonatal unit. *Arch Dis Child Fetal Neonatal Ed* 80(1):F64-8.

81. MacKenzie, F. M., Forbes K. J., Dorai-John T., Amyes S. G., and Gould I. M. 1997. Emergence of a carbapenem-resistant Klebsiella pneumoniae. *Lancet* 350(9080):783.

82. Huffman, J. A., Hull W. M., Dranoff G., Mulligan R. C., and Whitsett J. A. 1996. Pulmonary epithelial cell expression of GM-CSF corrects the alveolar proteinosis in GM-CSF-deficient mice. *J Clin Invest* 97(3):649-55.

83. Corti, M., Brody A. R., and Harrison J. H. 1996. Isolation and primary culture of murine alveolar type II cells. *Am J Respir Cell Mol Biol* 14(4):309-15.

84. Marsh, L. M., Cakarova L., Kwapiszewska G., von Wulffen W., Herold S., Seeger W., and Lohmeyer J. 2009. Surface expression of CD74 by type II alveolar epithelial cells: a potential mechanism for macrophage migration inhibitory factor induced-epithelial repair. *Am J Physiol Lung Cell Mol Physiol*.

85. Lowry, O. H., Rosebrough N. J., Farr A. L., and Randall R. J. 1951. Protein measurement with the Folin phenol reagent. *J Biol Chem* 193(1):265-75.

86. Steinmuller, M., Srivastava M., Kuziel W. A., Christman J. W., Seeger W., Welte T., Lohmeyer J., and Maus U. A. 2006. Endotoxin induced peritonitis elicits monocyte immigration into the lung: implications on alveolar space inflammatory responsiveness. *Respir Res* 7:30.

87. Herold, S., Steinmueller M., von Wulffen W., Cakarova L., Pinto R., Pleschka S., Mack M., Kuziel W. A., Corazza N., Brunner T., Seeger W., and Lohmeyer J. 2008. Lung epithelial apoptosis in influenza virus pneumonia: the role of macrophage-expressed TNF-related apoptosis-inducing ligand. *J Exp Med* 205(13):3065-77.

88. Li, C. M., Khosla J., Hoyle P., and Sannes P. L. 2001. Transforming growth factor-beta(1) modifies fibroblast growth factor-2 production in type II cells. *Chest* 120(1 Suppl):60S-61S.

89. Panos, R. J., Rubin J. S., Csaky K. G., Aaronson S. A., and Mason R. J. 1993. Keratinocyte growth factor and hepatocyte growth factor/scatter factor are heparin-binding growth factors for alveolar type II cells in fibroblast-conditioned medium. *J Clin Invest* 92(2):969-77.

90. Pogach, M. S., Cao Y., Millien G., Ramirez M. I., and Williams M. C. 2007. Key developmental regulators change during hyperoxia-induced injury and recovery in adult mouse lung. *J Cell Biochem* 100(6):1415-29.

91. Ray, P. 2005. Protection of epithelial cells by keratinocyte growth factor signaling. *Proc Am Thorac Soc* 2(3):221-5.

92. Aderem, A., and Ulevitch R. J. 2000. Toll-like receptors in the induction of the innate immune response. *Nature* 406(6797):782-7.

93. Cabanski, M., Steinmuller M., Marsh L. M., Surdziel E., Seeger W., and Lohmeyer J. 2008. PKR regulates TLR2/TLR4-dependent signaling in murine alveolar macrophages. *Am J Respir Cell Mol Biol* 38(1):26-31.

94. Gordon, S. 2003. Alternative activation of macrophages. *Nat Rev Immunol* 3(1):23-35.

References

95. Danto, S. I., Zabski S. M., and Crandall E. D. 1992. Reactivity of alveolar epithelial cells in primary culture with type I cell monoclonal antibodies. *Am J Respir Cell Mol Biol* 6(3):296-306.

96. Basseres, D. S., Levantini E., Ji H., Monti S., Elf S., Dayaram T., Fenyus M., Kocher O., Golub T., Wong K. K., Halmos B., and Tenen D. G. 2006. Respiratory failure due to differentiation arrest and expansion of alveolar cells following lung-specific loss of the transcription factor C/EBPalpha in mice. *Mol Cell Biol* 26(3):1109-23.

97. Chen, Z., Jin N., Narasaraju T., Chen J., McFarland L. R., Scott M., and Liu L. 2004. Identification of two novel markers for alveolar epithelial type I and II cells. *Biochem Biophys Res Commun* 319(3):774-80.

98. Williams, M. C., Cao Y., Hinds A., Rishi A. K., and Wetterwald A. 1996. T1 alpha protein is developmentally regulated and expressed by alveolar type I cells, choroid plexus, and ciliary epithelia of adult rats. *Am J Respir Cell Mol Biol* 14(6):577-85.

99. Tanimoto, A., Murata Y., Wang K. Y., Tsutsui M., Kohno K., and Sasaguri Y. 2008. Monocyte chemoattractant protein-1 expression is enhanced by granulocyte-macrophage colony-stimulating factor via Jak2-Stat5 signaling and inhibited by atorvastatin in human monocytic U937 cells. *J Biol Chem* 283(8):4643-51.

100. Guthridge, M. A., Stomski F. C., Thomas D., Woodcock J. M., Bagley C. J., Berndt M. C., and Lopez A. F. 1998. Mechanism of activation of the GM-CSF, IL-3, and IL-5 family of receptors. *Stem Cells* 16(5):301-13.

101. Sakamoto, K., Creamer B. A., Triplett A. A., and Wagner K. U. 2007. The Janus kinase 2 is required for expression and nuclear accumulation of cyclin D1 in proliferating mammary epithelial cells. *Mol Endocrinol* 21(8):1877-92.

102. Lawrence, T., Willoughby D. A., and Gilroy D. W. 2002. Anti-inflammatory lipid mediators and insights into the resolution of inflammation. *Nat Rev Immunol* 2(10):787-95.

103. Leslie, C. C., McCormick-Shannon K., Shannon J. M., Garrick B., Damm D., Abraham J. A., and Mason R. J. 1997. Heparin-binding EGF-like growth factor is a mitogen for rat alveolar type II cells. *Am J Respir Cell Mol Biol* 16(4):379-87.

104. Marshall, B. C., Xu Q. P., Rao N. V., Brown B. R., and Hoidal J. R. 1992. Pulmonary epithelial cell urokinase-type plasminogen activator. Induction by interleukin-1 beta and tumor necrosis factor-alpha. *J Biol Chem* 267(16):11462-9.

105. Burke, J. M. 1989. Stimulation of DNA synthesis in human and bovine RPE by peptide growth factors: the response to TNF-alpha and EGF is dependent upon culture density. *Curr Eye Res* 8(12):1279-86.

106. Fitzgerald, S. M., Chi D. S., Hall H. K., Reynolds S. A., Aramide O., Lee S. A., and Krishnaswamy G. 2003. GM-CSF induction in human lung fibroblasts by IL-1beta, TNF-alpha, and macrophage contact. *J Interferon Cytokine Res* 23(2):57-65.

107. Newton, R., Holden N. S., Catley M. C., Oyelusi W., Leigh R., Proud D., and Barnes P. J. 2007. Repression of inflammatory gene expression in human pulmonary epithelial cells by small-molecule IkappaB kinase inhibitors. *J Pharmacol Exp Ther* 321(2):734-42.

108. Lawrence, T., Gilroy D. W., Colville-Nash P. R., and Willoughby D. A. 2001. Possible new role for NF-kappaB in the resolution of inflammation. *Nat Med* 7(12):1291-7.

109. Mendez, M. P., Morris S. B., Wilcoxen S., Greeson E., Moore B., and Paine R., 3rd. 2006. Shedding of soluble ICAM-1 into the alveolar space in murine models of acute lung injury. *Am J Physiol Lung Cell Mol Physiol* 290(5):L962-70.

References

110. Braunstein, S., Kaplan G., Gottlieb A. B., Schwartz M., Walsh G., Abalos R. M., Fajardo T. T., Guido L. S., and Krueger J. G. 1994. GM-CSF activates regenerative epidermal growth and stimulates keratinocyte proliferation in human skin in vivo. *J Invest Dermatol* 103(4):601-4.

111. Bussolino, F., Ziche M., Wang J. M., Alessi D., Morbidelli L., Cremona O., Bosia A., Marchisio P. C., and Mantovani A. 1991. In vitro and in vivo activation of endothelial cells by colony-stimulating factors. *J Clin Invest* 87(3):986-95.

112. Sultan, A. S., Brim H., and Sherif Z. A. 2008. Co-overexpression of Janus kinase 2 and signal transducer and activator of transcription 5a promotes differentiation of mammary cancer cells through reversal of epithelial-mesenchymal transition. *Cancer Sci* 99(2):272-9.

113. Ballinger, M. N., Paine R., 3rd, Serezani C. H., Aronoff D. M., Choi E. S., Standiford T. J., Toews G. B., and Moore B. B. 2006. Role of granulocyte macrophage colony-stimulating factor during gram-negative lung infection with Pseudomonas aeruginosa. *Am J Respir Cell Mol Biol* 34(6):766-74.

114. Paine, R., 3rd, Preston A. M., Wilcoxen S., Jin H., Siu B. B., Morris S. B., Reed J. A., Ross G., Whitsett J. A., and Beck J. M. 2000. Granulocyte-macrophage colony-stimulating factor in the innate immune response to Pneumocystis carinii pneumonia in mice. *J Immunol* 164(5):2602-9.

115. Kitamura, Y., Hashimoto S., Mizuta N., Kobayashi A., Kooguchi K., Fujiwara I., and Nakajima H. 2001. Fas/FasL-dependent apoptosis of alveolar cells after lipopolysaccharide-induced lung injury in mice. *Am J Respir Crit Care Med* 163(3 Pt 1):762-9.

116. Zemans, R. L., Colgan S. P., and Downey G. P. 2009. Transepithelial migration of neutrophils: mechanisms and implications for acute lung injury. *Am J Respir Cell Mol Biol* 40(5):519-35.

117. Shen, L., Fahey J. V., Hussey S. B., Asin S. N., Wira C. R., and Fanger M. W. 2004. Synergy between IL-8 and GM-CSF in reproductive tract epithelial cell secretions promotes enhanced neutrophil chemotaxis. *Cell Immunol* 230(1):23-32.

118. Berclaz, P. Y., Carey B., Fillipi M. D., Wernke-Dollries K., Geraci N., Cush S., Richardson T., Kitzmiller J., O'Connor M., Hermoyian C., Korfhagen T., Whitsett J. A., and Trapnell B. C. 2007. GM-CSF regulates a PU.1-dependent transcriptional program determining the pulmonary response to LPS. *Am J Respir Cell Mol Biol* 36(1):114-21.

119. Branger, J., Knapp S., Weijer S., Leemans J. C., Pater J. M., Speelman P., Florquin S., and van der Poll T. 2004. Role of Toll-like receptor 4 in gram-positive and gram-negative pneumonia in mice. *Infect Immun* 72(2):788-94.

120. Schurr, J. R., Young E., Byrne P., Steele C., Shellito J. E., and Kolls J. K. 2005. Central role of toll-like receptor 4 signaling and host defense in experimental pneumonia caused by Gram-negative bacteria. *Infect Immun* 73(1):532-45.

9. Supplements

9.1. Materials and source of supply

[^{3}H]-thymidine	GE Healthcare, Germany
5x 1st strand buffer	Invitrogen, UK
Abbocath	Abbott, Germany
Acrylamide solution, Rotiphorese Gel 30	Roth, Germany
Agarose	Invitrogen, UK
Agarose, low-melting	Sigma-Aldrich, Germany
a-hamster-AlexaFluor 488 IgG	Invitrogen, UK
a-hamster-AlexaFluor 647 IgG	Invitrogen, UK
a-human Ki-67 PE mAb	BD Pharmingen, Germany
a-human pro-SP-C Ab	Chemicon International, UK
Ammonium persulfate (APS)	Promega, Germany
a-mouse Ki-67 mAb	Dako, Germany
a-mouse T1-α/podoplanin/gp36 mAb	Abcam, UK
a-mouse TNF-α mAb	R&D, Germany
a-mouse widespread cytokeratin Ab	Dako, Germany
Antibiotics (Pen/Strep)	PAA Laboratories, Austria
a-pSTAT5 Ab	Cell signalling, Germany
a-rabbit AlexaFluor 488 IgG	Invitrogen, UK
a-rabbit AlexaFluor 555 IgG	Invitrogen, UK
a-rabbit AlexaFluor 647 IgG	Invitrogen, UK
a-rabbit IgG horseradish peroxidase	Pierce, USA
a-rat AlexaFluor 488 IgG	Invitrogen, UK
a-STAT5 Ab	Cell signalling, Germany
Autoradiograph	(Amersham Hyperfilm ECL, GE Healthcare, Germany)
Biotinylated a-mouse CD16/32 mAb	BD Pharmingen, Germany
Biotinylated a-mouse CD31 mAb	BD Pharmingen, Germany
Biotinylated a-mouse CD45 mAb	BD Pharmingen, Germany
Bovine serum albumin (BSA)	Sigma-Aldrich, Germany
Bromophenol blue	Sigma-Aldrich, Germany

Supplements

Collagenase A	Roche, USA
DC protein assay	Bio-Rad, Germany
DifcoTM Skim Milk	BD Pharmingen, Germany
Dispase	BD Biosciences, Germany
Dithiothreitol (DTT)	Invitrogen, UK
DNAse	Serva, Germany
dNTPs	Roche, USA
Dulbecco's modified eagle medium (DMEM)	PAA Laboratories, Austria
E.coli lipopolysaccharide (0111:B4)	Calbiochem, Germany
ECL Plus Western Blotting Detection System	Amersham Biosciences, UK
EDTA	Biochrom, Germany
ELISA kits	R&D Systems, Germany
Ethanol	Riedel-de-Hän, Germany
Ethidium bromide solution	Carl Roth, Germany
Fc-Block	BD Pharmingen, Germany
Fetal Calf Serum (FCS)	PAA Laboratories, Austria
FITC-Albumin	Sigma-Aldrich, Germany
Glycine	Sigma-Aldrich, Germany
Goat IgG	R&D Systems, Germany
Hamster IgG	BD Pharmingen, Germany
Hank'S buffered saline solution (HBSS)	PAA laboratories, Austria
HEPES buffer	Invitrogen, UK
Hydrochloric acid (HCl)	Merck, Germany
Isoflurane (1-chloro-2,2,2-trifluoroethyl difluoromethyl ether)	Abbott, Germany
Ketavet (Ketamine hydrochloride)	Pharmacia & Upjohn, Germany
Matrigel	BD Biosciences, Germany
McConkey agar plates	Oxoid GmbH, Germany
Methanol	Fluka, Germany
M-MLV reverse transcriptase	Invitrogen, UK
Mounting medium with DAPI (Vectashield®)	Vector Laboratories, USA
Mouse IgG1 PE	BD Pharmingen, Germany
N,N,N',N'-tetramethyl-ethane-1.2-diamine (TEMED)	Sigma-Aldrich, Germany

Supplements

Pam3-Cys-Ser-Lys-Lys-Lys-Lys-OH (Pam$_3$CSK$_4$)	EMC Microcollections, Germany
Pappenheim staining solutions (May-Grünwald/Giemsa)	Merck, Germany
Paraformaldehyde (PFA)	Sigma-Aldrich, Germany
Phosphate buffered saline (PBS)	PAA Laboratories, Austria
Platinum Taq DNA polymerase	Invitrogen, UK
Platinum®SYBR®Green I qPCR SuperMix-UDG	Invitrogen, UK
Polyvinylidene difluoride (PVDF) membranes	Micron Separations, USA
Precision Plus Protein™ Standards	Bio-Rad, USA
Protease inhibitor cocktail	Roche, Germany
Rabbit IgG	Chemicon, Upstate
Random hexamers	Boehringer, Germany
Rat Collagen	R&D Systems, Germany
Rat IgG2a	BD Pharmingen, Germany
Recombinant murine TNF-α	R&D Systems, Germany
RNA isolation kit	Peqlab, Germany
RNase away	Molecular bioproducts, USA
RNase inhibitor	Promega, USA
RNeasy Mini Kit	Qiagen, Germany
Rompun (Xylazine hydrochloride)	Bayer, Germany
RPMI 1640 medium	PAA laboratories, Austria
Saponin	Calbiochem, Germany
Sodium chloride	Braun, Germany
Sodium dodecyl sulphate (SDS)	Sigma-Aldrich, Germany
Sodium ortho vanadate	Sigma-Aldrich, Germany
ß-mercaptoethanol	Sigma-Aldrich, Germany
Streptavidin linked APC-Cy7	BD Pharmingen, Germany
Streptavidin-linked Dynabeads® Paramagnetic particles	Invitrogen, UK
TissueTek OCT	Sakura Finetek, USA
Todd-Hewit Broth	BD Biosciences, Germany
Tris	Carl Roth, Germany

Trypan blue	Sigma-Aldrich, Germany
Trypsin	PAA laboratories, Austria
Tween 20	Sigma-Aldrich, Germany
Wildtype mice (C57/Bl6)	Charles River, Germany

9.2. Technical equipment and manufacturer

ABI PRISM 7900HT Sequence detector	Applied Biosystems, USA
Agilent Bioanalyser 2100	Agilent Tech., Germany
BioDocAnalyse video system	Whatman – Biometra, Germany
Cell culture incubator	Heraeus, Germany
Cell-culture plates/transwells: 24 wells	BD Labware, USA
Cell-culture plates: 48 wells	Greiner Bio-One, Germany
Chamber slides (8 well) Permanox®	Lab-Tek Thermofisher Scientific, Denmark
Cytospin Cytocentrifuge	Thermo Scientific, Germany
Developing machine, Curix 60	Agfa, Germany
Digital Imaging Software	Leica, Germany
Electrophoresis apparatus	Keutz, Germany
ELISA reader	Molecular Devices, Germany
Eppendorf tubes (0,6ml/1.5ml/2 ml)	Eppendorf, Germany
FACSCanto	BD, Germany
FACSDiva Software Package	BD, Germany
Filter tip	Greiner bio-one, Germany
Filter units	Millipore, USA
Fluorescence spectrophotometer	FL 880 microplate fluorescence reader, Bio-Tek Instruments, France
Light/Fluorescence microscope	Leica DM 2000 Light Microscope, Germany
Mini Protean 3 cell	Bio-Rad, USA
Mini spin centrifuge	Heraeus, Germany
Mini Trans Blot	Bio-Rad, USA
Multifuge centrifuge, 1S-R	Heraeus, Germany
NanoDrop ND-1000	Nano Technologies, USA

Supplements

PCR tubes (0.2 ml)	Applied Biosystems, USA
peqSTAR 96 Universal Gradient Cycler	Peqlab, Germany
Pipetmans: P10, P20, P100, P200, P1000	Gilson, France
Pipette tip	BD, Germany
Power supply	Biometra, Germany
Serological pipette: 5, 10, 25, 50 ml	Falcon, USA
Stereomicroscope	Leica MS5, Germany
Test tube thermostat	Roth, Germany
Test tubes :15, 50 ml	Greiner Bio-One, Germany
Vortex machine	Scientific Industries, Germany

9.3. List of primers for real-time RT-PCR

Gene Name	Forward primer sequence (5' → 3')	Reverse primer sequence (5' → 3')
C-EBPα	AAAGCCAAGAAGTCGGTGGAC	CTTTATCTCGGCTCTTGCGC
Cyclin D1	ACAGCTGCTTCGGGTCTGAGTTC	GGGAGCCACCTTCTTCTTTCA
FGF2	AGCGACCCACACGTCAAACT	CGTCCATCTTCCTTCATAGCAAG
GABRP	GCGCCTTGCTCAGTACACAA	ACGTTCCTCCGAAGCTCAAAT
GM-CSF	GAAGCATGTAGAGGCCATCA	GAATATCTTCAGGCGGGTCT
GM-CSFRß	TCCTTCCGGCCAGATAGTGA	GGAGCTGATGCTGACGTTCTT
GM-CSFRα	GCGACACGAGGATGAAGCA	CACTGCATACAGGAGCGCA
HMBS	GGTACAAGGCTTTCAGCATCGC	ATGTCCGGTAACGGCGGC
IGF-1	AGCTGGTGGATGCTCTTCAGTT	GGTGCCCTCCGAATGCT
KGF	TCGCACCCAGTGGTACCTG	ACTGCCACGGTCCTGATTTC
PDGFa	ATGCCAACCTCAGGAGAGAT	TGTCAGAAGCAGGTTCCTTG
PDGFb	CTGCTAGCGTCTGGTCA	CATCAAAGGAGCGGATGGAG
PDGFc	AATTGTGCCTGTTGTCTCCA	TATGCAATCCCTTGACTCCA
PDGFd	CCAGGACGGTCATTTACGAGA	GCGCTTCACCTCCACACAT
pro-SP-C	TCCTGATGGAGAGTCCACCG	CAGAGCCCCTACAATCACCAC
T1-α	ACAGGTGCTACTGGAGGGCTT	TCCTCTAAGGGAGGCTTCGTC
TGF-α	GGCTGCAGTGGTGTCTCA	AGCCACCACAGCCAGGA
TNFR1	TTCTGAGAGAAAGTGAGTGCGT	GGTTTGTGACATTTGCAAGC
TNFR2	AGGTCTGGAACCAGTTTCGT	CACACTCGGTTCTGCTGTTT
VEGF	TGTACCTCCACCATGCCAAGT	AATCGGACGGCAGTAGCTTC

10. Acknowledgements

I would like to acknowledge and extend my heartfelt gratitude to the many persons who have made the completion of this Dissertation possible.

First and foremost I wish to thank my supervisor Prof. Dr. Jürgen Lohmeyer for giving me the unique opportunity to join the lab and to begin my research carrier, for his vital support and encouragement throughout my PhD time, scientific discussions and helpful suggestions. Many thanks to my co-supervisor Dr. Susanne Herold, for being my major advisor and helped me to come up with my thesis topic, guided me over these years and provided many wise ideas for this dissertation. I would like to thank Prof. Dr. W. Seeger, Chairman and Director of the University of Giessen Lung Center, and the Department of Internal Medicine II, for his support, help and inspiration he extended.

I wish to thank my lab colleagues for providing a stimulating and fun environment in which to learn and grow, for the effort they invested to introduce me in every lab-technique and all the plentiful discussions. I am especially grateful to Leigh Marsh, Maciej Cabanski, Werner von Wullfen, Mirko Steinmüller, Zbigniew Zaslona and Katrin Högner. The technicians Petra Janssen and Dagmar Hensel are thanked for their invaluable help in many respects of my every-day lab work.

I am grateful to Dr. Oliver Eickelberg and Dr. Rory Morty for giving me the opportunity to join the International Program "Molecular Biology and Medicine of the Lung" (MBML) and for the excellent training they provided in lung biology.

Lastly, and most importantly, I am indebted to my parents, my brother, and my dear Vladimir. They supported me, encouraged me, taught me and loved me.

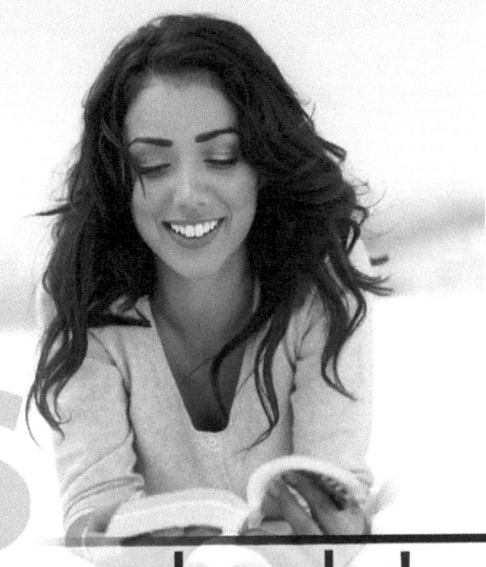

I want morebooks!

Buy your books fast and straightforward online - at one of the world's fastest growing online book stores! Environmentally sound due to Print-on-Demand technologies.

Buy your books online at
www.get-morebooks.com

Kaufen Sie Ihre Bücher schnell und unkompliziert online – auf einer der am schnellsten wachsenden Buchhandelsplattformen weltweit! Dank Print-On-Demand umwelt- und ressourcenschonend produziert.

Bücher schneller online kaufen
www.morebooks.de

OmniScriptum Marketing DEU GmbH
Heinrich-Böcking-Str. 6-8
D - 66121 Saarbrücken
Telefax: +49 681 93 81 567-9

info@omniscriptum.com
www.omniscriptum.com

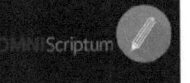

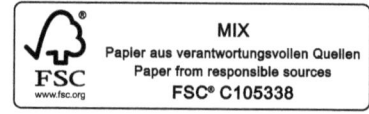

Printed by Books on Demand GmbH, Norderstedt / Germany